I0823042

Praise for *Moving Medicine Forward*

"In my work on the Blue Zones, I have identified many factors that have led to the longevity achieved by certain remarkable populations around the world. They include: a plant-based diet, physical activity such as gardening, social connections, a sense of purpose in life, and plenty of sleep. Let me now add one more suggestion that could add years to anyone's life: read Dr. Michael Klaper's wonderful explanation of nutrition and how medicine should be practiced: *Moving Medicine Forward*!"

—Dan Buettner, *New York Times* bestselling author and Emmy Award–winning producer of Netflix's *Live to 100: Secrets of the Blue Zones*

"In *Moving Medicine Forward*, Dr. Klaper delivers a strong prescription to doctors and patients alike: eating the right foods is a universal and science-informed approach for optimizing your health."

—William W. Li, MD, *New York Times* bestselling author of *Eat to Beat Disease* and *Eat to Beat Your Diet*

"Healthy cooking starts with an understanding of nutrition, and no book could help us understand nutrition more clearly and completely than *Moving Medicine Forward*."

—Carleigh Bodrug, *New York Times* bestselling author of *PlantYou* and *PlantYou Scrappy Cooking*

"Dr. Michael Klaper is a warm, caring human being who brings that empathy to his work as a physician and a half century of experience of using evidence-based nutrition to prevent, arrest, and even reverse disease—highly recommended!"

—Michael Greger, MD, FACLM, *New York Times* bestselling author of *How Not to Die* and *How Not to Diet*

"I have seen firsthand Dr. Klaper's integrity, brilliance, and unwavering dedication to his patients and to humanity. His message is clear: it's not only possible to move medicine forward—it's urgently necessary. This book points the way."

—Rip Esselstyn, #1 *New York Times* bestselling author of *Plant-Strong*

"Dr. Michael Klaper teaches an absolute master class in his brilliant book, *Moving Medicine Forward*. With more than five decades of experience as a practicing physician, Dr. Klaper has seen it all. He lays the foundation for the undeniable role that nutrition plays in our health. In analyzing how food matters, *Moving Medicine Forward* gets to the root of our society's health problems, providing framework and solutions enabling all of us to thrive."

—Robert Cheeke, *New York Times* bestselling coauthor of *The Plant-Based Athlete*

"Dr. Michael Klaper is one of the most trustworthy voices in nutrition, and writes with a level of honesty that's often missing from books published to attract sensation and promote diet wars. *Moving Medicine Forward* is a lesson in human nutrition and a guide for a healthier future grounded in evidence-based science. Thank you for this timely addition to my home library."

—Cyrus Khambatta, PhD, *New York Times* bestselling coauthor of *Mastering Diabetes*

"Almost everyone who has ever gone to a doctor knows that most doctors are not trained in nutrition. *Moving Medicine Forward* not only makes the case for nutritional education—it is nutritional education for doctors and the rest of us! Read this book to understand what foods to prepare for your meals, and what 'foods' to leave behind!"

—Kiki Nelson, national bestselling author of *Plantifully Lean* and *Plantifully Simple*

"Here is the headline for Dr. Michael Klaper's *Moving Medicine Forward*: Highly Experienced Medical Practitioner Tells What Must Be Told!"

—T. Colin Campbell, PhD,
Jacob Gould Schurman professor emeritus of nutritional biochemistry at Cornell University and international bestselling author of *The China Study*

"*Moving Medicine Forward* is a vitally important book whose time has come. For heart health, cancer prevention, reversing diabetes, and achieving the very best of health, the power of nutrition has been proven in research studies. Now, as doctors share this life-changing information with their patients, they will be giving them what may be the most powerful prescription of all."

—Neal D. Barnard, MD, FACC,
president of the Physicians Committee for Responsible Medicine and adjunct professor of medicine at George Washington University School of Medicine

"Dr. Michael Klaper is a legend. For decades, he has empowered his patients and the public to optimize their health through nutrition. He continues to travel the globe, teaching future doctors in medical schools how to empower their patients to achieve real health. He educates with facts delivered with earnestness, empathy, and compassion. And now his life's work can be in every person's home in this wonderful book. He is the truest example of a healer, and I am honored to call him my friend and to share his mission of challenging the status quo, bringing the truth about health to those who need it, and creating a healthier world."

—Brooke Goldner, MD, author of *Goodbye Lupus* and *Goodbye Autoimmune Disease*

"*Moving Medicine Forward* defines what can be the seismic revolution in health. Dr. Klaper clarifies how nutritional literacy for doctors, nurses, medical students, and the public will empower elimination of chronic illness and autoimmune diseases."

—Caldwell B. Esselstyn, Jr., MD,
author of *Prevent and Reverse Heart Disease*

"A compelling, sharply reasoned, and often witty wake-up call, *Moving Medicine Forward* challenges the medical establishment to accept the mounting evidence in favor of a plant-based diet—and to rethink how medicine is taught to the next generation of doctors. With clarity and conviction, it reveals how our food choices affect everything from personal health to planetary survival—and dares physicians to lead the way toward a more sustainable, evidence-based future."

—Ted Barnett, MD, FACLM, president of the Rochester Lifestyle Medicine Institute

"Dr. Michael Klaper is the kind of doctor children want to grow up to be: caring, curious, and creative. These attributes shine through *Moving Medicine Forward*, as Dr. Klaper shares with his colleagues and the rest of us a new way of seeing health—and the habits, attitudes, and food choices that promote it."

—Victoria Moran, author of *Main Street Vegan* and founder and director of Main Street Vegan Academy

"If there is one book you read on nutrition, this should be it. *Moving Medicine Forward* is the wake-up call that our society needs to right the ship and transform our collective health for the better."

—Dotsie Bausch, Olympic silver medal–winning cyclist and founder of Switch4Good

"Dr. Michael Klaper is a brilliant and steadfast pioneer in the fields of nutrition, health, and medicine. For decades, he has been a beacon of wisdom, compassion, and scientific clarity to all of us who have learned from and been inspired by his teachings in the plant-based community. It has been one of the greatest honors of my professional life to call him my mentor. With his compelling new book *Moving Medicine Forward*, Dr. Klaper's transformative message will reach even more people, empowering a global shift toward healing and conscious living."

—Julieanna (Hever) Risse, MS, RD, CPT, the Plant-Based Dietitian and author of *The Choose You Now Diet* and Idiot's Guides' *Plant-Based Nutrition*

"*Moving Medicine Forward* is a wake-up call, a road map, and a manifesto for the future of medicine. Dr. Michael Klaper's voice is bold, brilliant, and compassionate—as he shows how food is not just part of the problem, but the most powerful part of the solution. Michael Klaper is moving medicine—and humanity—forward. *Moving Medicine Forward* is pure gold. Every doctor, medical student, and human being who cares about health should read this book."

—Ocean Robbins, cofounder and CEO of Food Revolution Network and author of *31-Day Food Revolution*

"Dr. Klaper's voice is a clarion call for medicine to return to its highest purpose: to heal, to prevent, and to empower. With clarity, compassion, and nutritional integrity, he urges us to move medicine forward—beyond symptom suppression and into a new paradigm of restoration, renewal, and enduring health."

—Brenda Davis, RD, plant-based author and trailblazer

"In *Moving Medicine Forward*, Dr. Michael Klaper pulls back the curtain on one of the greatest shortcomings in modern medicine—our neglect of nutrition—and lays out a compelling path toward a more informed, prevention-focused, plant-predominant future. This is essential reading for physicians, trainees, and anyone who believes that food should once again be part of the prescription."

—Kim Allan Williams, Sr., MD, MACC, FAHA, MASNC, FESC

"In *Moving Medicine Forward*, Dr. Michael Klaper shares a paradigm of hope and empowerment that has the potential to transform medicine. Drawing on his years of professional experience, as well as a strong body of scientific research, he demonstrates with clarity and compassion the power of nutrition to help us move beyond treating symptoms, to preventing and even reversing many of the chronic diseases of our time. While acknowledging the very real forces that often stand in the way of nutritional and lifestyle medicine becoming more widespread, Dr. Klaper offers a powerful road map to truly move medicine forward. This book is a must-read for anyone who wants to experience and empower others toward a path of greater health and wellness."

—Angela Crawford, PhD, psychologist, plant-based educator, and author of *The Vegan Transformation*

"Few people combine medical expertise with genuine kindness like Dr. Michael Klaper. His dedication to helping others live healthier, more compassionate lives is truly inspiring, and comes across in the pages of *Moving Medicine Forward*."

—Chef AJ, author, YouTube host, and vegan since 1977

"Dr. Michael Klaper's *Moving Medicine Forward* is a groundbreaking guide that reimagines the future of healthcare through the power of nutrition. It has been a long wait for a book from this icon, but as both a patient and the host of one of the world's most popular nutrition podcasts, I've seen firsthand how his wisdom and compassion transform lives. This inspiring book belongs in the hands of every physician, patient, and anyone who believes medicine should truly heal."

—Chuck Carroll, host of
the Physicians Committee for Responsible Medicine's
The Exam Room Podcast

"In this compelling book, Dr. Michael Klaper sets the stage for a healthier society by prioritizing the role that nutrition plays in wellness. Health starts with the foods we eat. Dr. Klaper argues forcefully that physicians need to understand this. *Moving Medicine Forward* is not just a book title or a novel concept; it's a paradigm shift and the start of a health revolution. Read this book and join the effort to move medicine forward."

—Dr. James F. Loomis, medical director at Barnard Medical Center,
cohost of *The Doc and Chef*,
and featured in the documentary *The Game Changers*

"As a longtime mentor, friend, and now colleague, Dr. Klaper helped shape my approach to clinical practice early in my career, offering invaluable advice and guidance on tough patient cases. I witnessed his passion for incorporating nutrition into medicine firsthand, and that same passion shines through in this book, which will no doubt inspire readers to recognize the powerful role of diet in health."

—Dr. Matthew Nagra, doctor of naturopathic medicine

"*Moving Medicine Forward* is more than a book—it's a mirror held up to modern medicine and a compass pointing us home. Dr. Klaper reminds us that healing isn't found solely in high-tech tools or prescriptions, but in the simplest, most profound of places: our choices, our compassion, and our connection to food. He calls on us—as clinicians and as people—to return to the roots of medicine and to reimagine healthcare with heart, purpose, and integrity. This book will lead the way."

—Columbus Batiste, MD, FACC, FSCAI,
author of *Selfish: A Cardiologist's Guide to Healing a Broken Heart*

"*Moving Medicine Forward* distills timeless wisdom, rigorous science, and decades of clinical experience into an antidote for chronic disease and burnout—reigniting passion and vision for healthcare professionals everywhere. A must-read for clinicians and a hope-filled guide for patients, Dr. Michael Klaper's long-awaited book is a rare gift that empowers us to heal, lead, and truly move medicine forward."

—Scott Stoll, MD, FABPMR, cofounder of The Plantrician Project and Olympian

"Dr. Michael Klaper is one of the kindest people I've ever met. He brings to *Moving Medicine Forward* the same decency, warmth, humor, and compassion that have made him a hero to so many of us who want humanity to view animals as friends, not food."

—Gene Baur, cofounder and president of Farm Sanctuary and author of *Living the Farm Sanctuary Life*

"What I love about *Moving Medicine Forward* is the hope in it. Dr. Klaper shows how a whole food, plant-based lifestyle isn't some fringe idea—it's real science that can stop heart disease, diabetes, and so many of the things we've been told are 'just part of aging.' It's proof that it's never too late to turn things around."

—Jeremy LaLonde, host of the *PB with J* podcast

MOVING MEDICINE FORWARD

What More Doctors Should Know About Nutrition—and How It Can Save Your Life

Michael Klaper, MD

with Glen Merzer

BenBella Books, Inc.
Dallas, TX

To students of medicine, everywhere.

BenBella Books, Inc.
8080 N. Central Expressway
Suite 1700
Dallas, TX 75206
benbellabooks.com
Send feedback to feedback@benbellabooks.com

BenBella is a federally registered trademark.

Printed in the United States of America
10 9 8 7 6 5 4 3 2 1

Library of Congress Control Number: 2025044594
ISBN 9781637748268 (hardcover)
ISBN 9781637748275 (electronic)

Editing by Rick Chillot
Copyediting by Scott Calamar
Proofreading by Mary White and Cheryl Beacham
Indexing by WordCo Indexing Services
Text design and composition by Jordan Koluch
Illustrations by Bruce Sachs
Cover design by Morgan Carr
Printed by Lake Book Manufacturing

Contents

INTRODUCTION

To be a physician is the privilege of a lifetime. What can be more rewarding than to help others heal? Medicine allows me to attend to humanity at its most vulnerable, to bear witness to both the fragility and the resilience of the human spirit, and to participate in the miraculous process of healing.

As a medical doctor, I am routinely admitted intimately into the lives of people from all walks of life, even if only for a brief period of time. With each encounter, I learn from my patients, and they learn from me, as we navigate together the various challenges that life inevitably presents to their health.

Often, my work has involved relatively simple medical craft, to set a fractured bone or drain an abscess, thus altering the structure or function of the body to stop the pain, promote healing, and, hopefully, vanquish the disease process. I take as much pride in doing the fundamental procedures as I do in trying to steer a seriously ill patient along a rocky road back to health.

But the practice of medicine, I have learned, is not only about curing diseases. On the deepest level, it is about meeting people where they are, and walking with them on their path. As physicians, sometimes we heal, sometimes we comfort, and sometimes we simply bear witness. It is all service to our fellow humans, and that, at its core, is why I became a doctor.

It has been a high honor to be invited into people's private, precious, unique life journeys. I have felt that honor uninterruptedly in a medical career that has now lasted fifty-three years—with no end in sight. I intend to practice for as long as I can do so effectively.

Simply put, I love my profession.

I am also, at this moment, profoundly embarrassed by it.

How could I not be embarrassed, as I watch what seems to be the willful ignorance of the medical establishment result in the grim public health wreckage we see all around us: a population grown comfortable with normalized obesity and accustomed to skyrocketing rates of type 2 diabetes, a tsunami of lethal heart attacks and strokes, and ever more lethal colon cancers that are now especially afflicting the young. Ours is a population traumatized by rising deaths from opioids and suicide. It is a population with ten times the maternal mortality rate of other high-income nations. Despite ingesting staggering amounts of powerful, pricey pharmaceutical drugs each day, our population still suffers, by far, the worst health outcomes of any wealthy country on our planet. Our longevity remains unimpressive; we live about four fewer years, on average, than those in comparable countries, while spending almost twice as much on healthcare.[1] By any reasonable quality-of-life metric, we fall woefully short.

This is our medical report card. There is no escaping the fact that the miserable state of America's public health reflects poorly on us—the medical profession. We have been, at best, passive observers of a series of catastrophic declines in the health of the people we serve. At worst, we have accelerated those declines. We cannot wash our hands of this tragic record.

We doctors have failed America terribly, and we have done so with stunning, almost criminal negligence. We have the capacity to reverse disease, and yet we run from it. We have the tools to increase longevity, but we leave them in the toolbox. We can show our patients how to markedly improve their health and the quality of their lives, yet we deem our patients incapable of utilizing this information. Incredibly, and most bafflingly, we often refuse to learn and utilize this information ourselves.

Yes, we are skilled at applying lifesaving care in emergency rooms to patients suffering acute medical crises. We can and do demonstrate those skills with courage, determination, and dedication on a daily basis in hospitals and urgent care centers across this country. We are a match for any doctors on the planet in saving the lives of those who have suffered terrible injuries, need intricate surgeries to remove brain tumors, or are in the midst of cardiac arrest. We are well trained for crisis medicine.

But we are caught humiliatingly flat-footed should our day-in, day-out patients ask us for commonsense health advice in the hope of staying out of those very same emergency rooms.

For patients who want to lose weight, stop a slide towards type 2 diabetes, protect their hearts, reverse inflammatory conditions, or improve their blood pressure—in short, to become healthy—conventional Western medicine has virtually nothing to offer beyond an array of potent pills that usually can do no more than control symptoms, while often generating more harm than good, and certainly do not reverse the underlying disease states. Collectively, we physicians dismiss the subject of "health" entirely, as if it's a subject more fit for self-styled wellness coaches, supplement purveyors, or shamans—as if it's irrelevant to our profession, which too many of my colleagues see as concerning only the diagnosis and treatment of disease.

That is a shockingly narrow view of a powerful and noble calling.

It's high time that we stop acting as a feckless profession, given that so many of our sick and bereft patients, in understandable desperation, place in us their hope, trust, and respect—and even their lives. At this point, I feel that we are treated with more admiration than we deserve, given our collective report card when it comes to safeguarding public health. The moment now demands that we start practicing evidence-based medicine that takes the patient's daily physiology into account, which inevitably means taking the patient's daily diet into account. Only that way can we deliver the level of true healing that our patients deserve.

Then, at last, physicians can truly earn the deference and respect that we are now generally afforded.

Chapter One

ETIOLOGY UNKNOWN?

I never had any desire to stray from the well-marked, time-honored path to a conventional medical career that promised so much in the way of both material and nonmaterial rewards.

That I would become a doctor was never much in question. There appears to be a knack for biology in my genes. My father was a dentist, with his own practice on the South Side of Chicago. He went into dentistry surely, in part, to make a living, and in part to relieve people's pain—but I think largely because he was so fascinated by the anatomical miracle of teeth and the complex and dynamic world that exists within our mouths. My mother was a lab technician who did manual blood counts under a microscope for Cook County Hospital. My brother became a high school biology teacher, and one of his daughters is now the dean in the School of Freshwater Sciences at the University of Wisconsin. I grew enamored with biology mainly as a consequence of idyllic childhood summers spent on a dairy farm.

In the late 1940s and 1950s, fearsome polio epidemics rolled through the major cities every summer, leaving some children with paralyzed limbs and others able to breathe only while entrapped in an iron lung. This was terrifying, naturally. But it was also, for a child like me, an early lesson in the centrality of health in human experience. To shield my brother and me from this scourge, my parents would whisk us off to spend summers on the farm of my mother's crusty Uncle Charlie. The day after the spring school semester ended, the family would usually hop into the car, or occasionally pile onto a train—the Flambeau 400 streamliner—for the six-hour ride to Elcho, Wisconsin, in the northern part of the state. There, Uncle Charlie owned three hundred acres of dense northern forests, having cleared about one-third of the trees to open land for a dairy operation and a mink "farm."

And so I spent the first fourteen summers of my life immersed in nature, waking up at 6 AM to start the day, milking cows as soon as I was old enough, stacking hay bales, cleaning out the chicken coops, and driving tractors—a skill I was taught, strange as it may seem, at the age of nine. Those summers, filled with clear blue skies, punctuated by majestic afternoon thunderstorms, and animated by songbirds and butterflies, were pure magic to me. The natural world reigned everywhere, the streams teeming with fish, turtles, and frogs, the sky alive with soaring hawks and darting golden finches, the land host to foxes, deer, chipmunks, squirrels, raccoons, skunks, groundhogs, wild hogs, and more—and then of course there were all the animals owned by Uncle Charlie that were being raised for milking, skinning, and slaughter to provide food and clothing for us clever humans. There were companion animals as well—the cats and dogs that seemed to enjoy the farm as much as I did. Cicadas and crickets sang through the night. Biology was a Technicolor summer symphony all around me, a stark contrast to the black-and-white Chicago winters.

Of course, when there was no farmwork to be done, my brother, three cousins, and I would play. We horsed around a good deal, jumping from bale forts in haylofts, and clambering over farm equipment in the sheds, so naturally plenty of injuries arose. If someone got cut or bruised, I was the one in the group who wanted to tend to the person, to apply the Band-Aid, to administer the aspirin, to make sure he or she was okay. That impulse to help heal people got married to my love of biology and of the natural world, and so the goal of becoming a physician animated me from such a young age that I cannot remember a time when it did not.

I took physics and chemistry in high school and loved the insights they revealed, helping me more and more to make sense of the natural world. I began to understand that the same kind of chemical reactions that took place in humans also took place in cows and bears and fish and are all subject to the same laws of physics, chemistry, and biology. All converge into the wonder of life. A future physician, I came to believe, need only learn the laws of science and then apply them to one's patients with skill and empathy—surely that wouldn't be too hard to do.

As a pre-med undergraduate at the University of Illinois Urbana, I majored in zoology, minored in astronomy and psychology, and took an elective course in human anatomy that was pure poetry to me. I relished learning the ancient, beautifully descriptive names of each muscle, bone, and nerve. How can one not love a science that describes the muscle that bends the small, fifth finger as the *flexor digiti minimi*? After receiving the blessed acceptance letter in the spring of 1968, I headed off to medical school at the Chicago Medical Center of the University of Illinois at the tender age of twenty.

I was the model student, never a boat-rocker or hell-raiser; I was there to absorb information, to learn the tools of my craft. Other than being a year or two younger than most of my classmates, I did not in any way deviate from the norm. Mostly I worked alone, letting the elegant, powerful fundamentals of biochemistry, physiology, and pathology flow from textbook pages and lab experiences into my understandings of the workings of the human body. Occasionally, when exams were coming up, I joined study groups, where I made friends and discussed the pros and cons of different specialties with my classmates. We weighed potential careers over meals of lamb and beef in many Greek restaurants in the neighborhood. (I remember thinking then of vegetarians as some kind of strange outliers.) Disciplined and determined, I had no intention of following a career path that would differ in any significant way from that of any of my medical school peers. It was just a matter of selecting the medical specialty that suited my skills and personality the best.

During the last quarter of my fourth year of medical school, as an elective course, I spent a dozen long nights—from seven in the evening till seven in the morning—in the trauma unit of the famous Cook County Hospital, the model for the setting of the TV show *ER*. I was available to help if needed, but mainly I was there to observe how a trauma unit functions; I felt like an auditor in a class on mayhem. Those emotionally exhausting nights were a bracing lesson in the capacity of human beings to do violence to one another. I saw things that I will never unsee, though I certainly wish I could. I saw more bullet wounds and knife wounds in two weeks than any doctor should need to witness in a career.

I remember becoming physically nauseated after witnessing what had happened to a woman who was transported into our ER. She had been assaulted by her jealous boyfriend with a baseball bat; he had hit her so hard in the head that her face, now a deep purple from the venous blood oozing from her fractured facial bones into the skin, had become untethered from her skull. This had left her with what's known as a *Le Fort IV fracture*, meaning that all four bony points of connection of the face to the skull were severed. I watched the surgeon try to reposition her face, moving it first to one side, then to the other, so that it could be surgically reattached. I wondered what could be in any human being's heart that such unthinkable violence could be inflicted upon another human being—and, in this case, to a person with whom the assailant had been intimate.

Whether this experience in the trauma unit of Cook County Hospital helped inform my future career as a doctor I cannot say, but it had a profound effect on me as a human being. As I left my nights in the trauma unit behind, I became committed to living a life of nonviolence, of dynamic harmlessness—living in a way that does the most good and the least harm—so that if there was ever any hint of fury or resentment in my heart, I could identify it and extinguish it. I wanted no trace of violence in my life—not verbally, not mentally, and certainly not physically. I began reading the writings of Martin Luther King Jr., Mahatma Gandhi, and Nelson Mandela. I admired all three men for their courage, for their dedication to nonviolence, and for their humility.

At that juncture I also admired, I will admit, another and manifestly lesser example of humility: the humility of my profession. Yes, I say humility, because throughout my years in med school, two words arose often, both in textbooks and on the lips of my professors: *"Etiology Unknown."* This was a fancy way of saying that the cause of a given disease had not yet been determined by science. We studied, for example, the symptoms of heart disease, and the pharmacological and surgical treatments for that number one killer of Americans. And what turned out to be the cause of the gruel-like plaques building up on the inner walls of the heart's arteries, blocking blood flow and killing the patient? *"Etiology Unknown."*

We studied hypertension (high blood pressure), a veritable plague in our society that causes strokes, heart failure, kidney disease, and blindness, and tends to afflict people as they age. We learned how to determine which drugs to employ to gradually (or quickly) bring a patient's high blood pressure down to safer levels. The cause of high blood pressure? Good old *"Etiology Unknown."*

We studied autoimmune diseases, like *lupus erythematosus*, a maddeningly diverse but related set of conditions that have in common the puzzling fact that the patient's robust immune system has begun attacking their own cells. I was surely not surprised to learn that such a complex and befuddling disease was another case of *"Etiology Unknown."*

It was perhaps a bit unnerving that so many diseases had unknown causes, but at the very least you had to hand it to the profession for bravely owning up to what it did not know. I took it as a sign of integrity.

As my career in medicine progressed, I began to realize that *"Etiology Unknown"* was not merely an expression of humility. There was an implicit promise of progress attendant to it. You could stitch together that promise from any number of comments made by our professors; essentially, they took this form:

While the etiology of cardiovascular disease may be unknown today, there are legions of top-notch research scientists studying the issue night and day in laboratories around our great nation. Look to the geneticists and in particular to the molecular biochemists to soon achieve a whole new world of breathtaking discoveries that will remake medicine, opening up shining new vistas in medical care. Do not bet against these medical sleuths! Surely, one day soon, the etiology of all these perplexing conditions will be determined and effective treatments derived for every one of them. Trust in science!

You couldn't help but be impressed. My professors, accomplished scientists that they were, readily acknowledged what they did not know, but they had utter faith that the principles of science, applied rigorously, would before long unlock such mysteries as the etiology of cardiovascular disease, to which an answer could not come too soon, given that hundreds of thousands of our countrymen were falling prey to these confounding conditions every year. I was proud to be joining a discipline that was at once humble and ambitious.

I kept my head down, became an MD at the age of twenty-four, and headed off to Vancouver, BC, to begin my long-dreamed-of career in medicine. Upon finishing my one year of medical internship at Vancouver General Hospital, I was invited to join a busy general practice in a suburban community near Vancouver.

It was not without a heavy dose of optimism and a significant degree of pride that I accepted this position. I would be working with three very accomplished senior physicians. My name would be on the door alongside theirs. I would earn a very respectable salary. At the tender age of twenty-five, I was no longer a med student or an intern or a resident—I was now a working physician, determined that my practice of medicine would be looked upon favorably by my more experienced and accomplished colleagues.

I was also, to be honest, a bit nervous about it. My patients, I knew, were not going to cut me any slack because I was young and inexperienced, nor should they. My greatest fear was the thought of missing a diagnosis.

After all, if I didn't recognize a rare condition, something like *Brugada syndrome* (a potentially life-threatening heart arrhythmia) or *adrenoleukodystrophy* (a genetic condition that damages nerve cells), my negligence could lead to a patient's suffering—or even death. I certainly didn't want to live with that on my conscience.

Deep inside, I felt a bit like an imposter. My conscious mind told me that I was trained and ready, but my unconscious mind was hardly convinced. On my first morning of medical practice, the fears were building: *They're going to bring sick people in here! Some of them are going to need a doctor! Where do I find one in this town?*

To choke down that immobilizing feeling of insecurity, I phoned the chief medical resident at Vancouver General Hospital, under whom I had recently trained, and unburdened myself of my insecurities.

"Listen, Michael," he said. "You're in North America. When you hear hoofbeats, don't look for zebras. It's going to be horses."

I knew he was right. In daily suburban medical practice, I was most often going to be seeing the same ordinary complaints: infections, injuries, and common degenerative diseases. Rarely would I run into a "zebra" with some rare and extraordinary condition that required a uniquely insightful diagnosis.

"Come on, Michael, you know how to do this," my friend/mentor said to me. "You understand the essence of how to practice medicine. Your patient comes in, you take the medical history, do a physical exam, order your labs—by the time you do all that, the odds are overwhelming that you'll know what you are looking at and what to do. It becomes obvious. If your patient reports to you that he smokes two packs a day, he's got shaking chills and a fever, he's sweaty and coughing up green guck, and through your stethoscope you hear his lungs sounding like a boiler factory—he's clearly got pneumonia, with bacteria and pus spreading through his lung tissue. In short, if you just shut up and really listen to your patient and their body, they'll usually *tell you* the diagnosis. And if you keep on listening, they'll usually tell you what treatment they need!"

He was, of course, absolutely right. Looking back now on fifty-three years of practice, I can say that I've seen very few zebras. Instead, I've seen the same, all-too-common, lumbering herd of Western diseases over and over again: obesity, hypertension, type 2 diabetes, inflammatory conditions, cardiovascular disease, fatty liver disease, and cancer of many organs in the body.

There was something different, though, about the patients I began to see in my medical office compared to the patients I had seen in Chicago and Vancouver hospitals during my training. These new patients, for the most part, were not suffering acute medical crises. I had been trained on hospital patients who were very sick; now I was seeing patients who were developing conditions—hypertension, diabetes or prediabetes, angina (chest pain from clogged heart arteries)—that might send them to the hospital one day if unchecked, but for now, in my office, they did not think of themselves as "sick." They were, in effect, patients who were coming for wellness checks or to report mild symptoms. My job was to help them improve their health, steer them clear of disease, prevent or stall declines in function of their vital organs, and keep them out of the emergency room; there was no urgent need to save their lives or limbs.

That may sound as if my task would be an easy one, but though I was well prepared for crisis medicine, I was hardly prepared for the more pressing task that now faced me: how to stop my patients' slides towards a medical catastrophe and help them start on an upward trajectory towards true health. When I started the job, I didn't recognize my inadequacy at this task, but after a few months it became clear.

Here's what would happen. The patient would enter the office and register at the front desk. The nurse, armed with a list of patients to be seen that day, would call the patient's name, escort the patient into the exam room, sit them down, record their chief complaint that had brought them to the office, and take their vital signs. All of that information would be written on the patient's chart, which would then be deposited in the wooden chart holder on the outside of the exam room door.

I would lift that chart up out of the rack before entering the office and review it. And I would read that Mrs. Smith, who had last come to the office a few months ago at 220 pounds, had now reached 240 pounds with a cholesterol level to match. Beyond those formidable numbers, now she was developing chest pains, frequent urination, and sleep apnea. I didn't want to open the door, didn't want to see Mrs. Smith; I had nothing to offer her. Should I tell her to stop eating so much? To try to walk a little more? I knew she didn't want to hear that kind of advice. Should I increase the dosages of her cholesterol medications? Or switch her to a different cholesterol drug? The woman had clearly lost control of her health; now she was my problem. What the hell could I do for her? I would put on a brave face and enter the room. I would spend the appointment time listening and empathizing, making bland suggestions and ordering more tests—and feeling like an imposter the whole time.

The next patient might be someone with type 2 diabetes who was already insulin dependent. I had raised his insulin dosage a month ago, and now, according to his labs, with his hemoglobin A1c (HgbA1c, a measure of blood sugar over the last two to three months) climbing from 7.4% to 7.7%, showing him walking around with an average blood sugar of 171 mg/dL, it looked like I would need to raise it again. I didn't know anything about what brought on insulin resistance (its etiology, after all, was unknown); I just knew that this poor guy seemed to have an evil spirit dwelling in his body called *type 2 diabetes* that voraciously devoured the already obscene amounts of insulin that I had prescribed and he had injected, leaving him with blood sugar levels that rarely dipped into the normal range.

The patient who followed, another regular, would be suffering headaches, perhaps related to his ever-increasing blood pressure. How many times could I increase his beta-blocker and alpha methyldopa medications before he would start experiencing side effects? Potentially serious ones, such as lowering his heart rate so severely (bradycardia) that he passes out while driving on the highway? Or should I try different drugs altogether?

He had a nasty reaction to the previous two BP medications I had prescribed, with pounding heartbeat, flush face, and nausea lasting for hours.

I would read the charts of patient after patient before opening the door, and my heart would sink—multiple times a day. *Lupus? Hell, I don't want to write another script for prednisone—these lupus patients keep getting more and more obese and diabetic from that drug. Rheumatoid arthritis? I have nothing to offer these patients except referral to a rheumatologist. Heartburn and hiatal hernia? Send them to the gastroenterologist—let them be her problem. Angina? I'll send that one to the cardiologist. A bad cough? Send her to the pulmonologist!*

I sent one patient after another to specialists. I told myself that these medical punts would benefit the patient, but they left me feeling impotent and frustrated. Had I become nothing more than a triage officer and errand boy for the specialists in town?

Finally, I'd pick up a chart with some good news. A patient was in my exam room with a gash on his arm. *Yes! I could fix a laceration! I knew how to do that!* I would numb the skin with lidocaine, clean the cut with iodine (I would never do that today[1]), sew it up with sutures, clean the area a final time, and dress the wound. Yay! At last, a medical victory I could honestly feel good about!

Oh, how I hungered for lacerations to repair, abscesses to drain, and foreign bodies to remove from eyes, ears, and under the skin. Nosebleeds were welcome, too. I could cauterize those and stop the frightening flow of blood, much to the relief of the patient—and me!

Learning that a patient with an ear infection was waiting for me I took as relatively good news; these infections were easy to diagnose, and they usually responded well to oral or topical antibiotics. Sprains and all kinds of physical injuries also made for satisfying visits; I enjoyed chatting with my injury-prone patients, whom I appreciated more than they could know for the very reason that they presented problems that were fixable.

Unfortunately, the obese, wheezing, hypertensive, diabetic patients kept shuffling into my office with ever-worsening metabolic disorders;

they became the bane of my practice. They were a living rebuke to my high opinion of myself as a doctor. I kept increasing their dosages of medicines, and with extraordinary ingratitude, they kept growing sicker and sicker. My only recourse was to refer them to specialists, as I was trained to do, and thus rid myself of the burden of dealing with them.

After almost five years of general practice, my days in the office began to fall into worrisome ruts. Repeating patterns of climbing weights and increasing blood sugar and cholesterol levels painted most every patient's chart. Monthly visits from these same patients turned into dreary episodes of fretting over worsening symptoms, furrowing my brow over ominous lab results, then writing prescriptions for stronger medications designed to, at best, delay some metabolic disaster.

All my clinical decisions were conventional and squarely defensible as "standard of care." My drug-based treatments were validated and reinforced by most every published study I read in the scientific journals on my desk—and by each speaker whose words enlightened me at medical conferences. As far as I could tell, I was practicing medicine as well as any of my colleagues.

That was little comfort. We were *all* failing our patients.

Despite my earnest efforts and my applications of the latest approved therapies, I would regularly get the dreaded call from the cardiologist in the hospital emergency room informing me that "Your patient Mary just had a major myocardial infarction," or "We have your patient Joe here—it looks like he had a nasty stroke." My patients were suffering medical catastrophes, and I felt powerless to protect them.

And so, as the early years in practice rolled by, I found that large chunks of my clinical time were being spent bailing these folks out of dire straits with heroic measures when their chronic diseases turned acute. Midnight encounters in the ER to spar with tight, asthmatic lungs that were choking out their owner's breath, or to subdue runaway high blood pressure that could blow out a cerebral artery—well, that made for exciting medicine, to be sure, but I knew I was just putting out fires. These experiences began to resemble the crisis medicine in which I had been expertly trained at medical school, with one significant difference: *I knew these people.* They had been my patients before the crises erupted, and I had failed to forestall these emergencies that increasingly came to feel inevitable.

Crisis medicine proved distinctly less rewarding to practice when I felt implicated in the crisis.

Eventually, I came to feel like a medical fraudster each time I welcomed a new patient into my office, knowing full well that I could not protect them against the diseases most likely to kill them. I began to face each day's full schedule of patients with unrelenting dread.

I had another reason to be concerned. As a young bachelor, my own diet consisted of fast foods: fried chicken, cheeseburgers, and a steady stream of standard fare at local Asian, Indian, and Mexican restaurants. I'd put on weight, gaining thirty pounds. My blood pressure mounted a steady march northward, reliably holding in the 148/88 mm Hg range.

When I visited home, my father could no longer walk very far with ease. He suffered from intermittent claudication—obstructed blood flow in the arteries of his legs. He was starting to get angina pains as well; it only made sense that the same arterial disease that was affecting his legs would naturally affect the arteries supplying his heart.

I knew that I had his genes. I knew that it was likely that, probably in only a couple of decades' time, I would begin to develop the same metabolic disorders that were bringing on the inexorable decline of my father and of so many of my patients in Vancouver.

It just seemed to be a fact of life that as people got older, they generally got fatter and sicker, and I seemed to be one of those people. It was a depressing thought.

After almost five years of this intense, increasingly discouraging primary care practice, a favorite patient of mine suffered a severe stroke. He was a generous, witty, sixty-four-year-old man who was a linguistics professor at one of Vancouver's universities. In his visits to my office, I had so enjoyed his clever and colorful stories from his extensive travels. He was yet another patient whose bloodwork seemed to get a little worse with each visit. On the day of his stroke, he was reduced to a mute, hemiplegic hulk of a man, unable to speak, swallow, or change his own underwear. This good man was an innocent victim of *Etiology Unknown,* a diabolical foe from which I could not save him. When I witnessed him in that state, I felt I could no longer continue with this ongoing deception.

These people deserved a real doctor. I was an imposter.

Battered by my early failure as a physician and frustrated by the reality that I was doing little more than sending patient after patient off to see specialists who, at least theoretically, might be able to help them more than I could, I hit upon a potential solution that makes little sense to me now and therefore presents a challenge to explain. But here, for what it's worth, was my solution: *I would practice frontier medicine!* I would find some isolated spot in Canada or the States where a severe shortage of medical care existed and set up shop, or join the practice of, at most, one or two other physicians. There would be no specialists around to whom I could refer folks, so I would no longer feel like an errand boy for the specialists. Effectively, I would have to be, for my patients, almost every type of specialist—by becoming a general practitioner so well-rounded and skilled that actual specialists would not be required.

What in the world made me believe that I would have greater success helping patients if there were few other doctors around? I don't have a solid answer to that glaringly obvious question, beyond the excuse that I was young and foolish. Clearly, I had a desire to return to a rustic setting like the one I had cherished for so many summers as a boy. And maybe there was one other factor at play: I may have believed that, in preparing to meet the challenge of becoming a general practitioner sufficiently well rounded and skilled as to obviate the need for specialists, I might improve my performance as a doctor. I might not dread seeing my patients if I could learn what to do for them. This was a path, after all, that would force upon me a good deal of continuing education. In any case, surely having one doctor in an isolated area would be a lot better than having none, or having three doctors would be considerably better than having two, so I could be confident that my service would present some benefit to an underserved population.

After I undertook additional training in several medical specialties at university-affiliated hospitals in Vancouver (including a six-month traineeship in anesthesia, six months of general surgery, three months of chest surgery, three months of plastic surgery, and three months of orthopedics to learn early fracture care) and six months of obstetrics at the University of California at San Francisco, where I delivered almost two hundred babies, a doctor friend mentioned that there was a clinic looking for a weekend doc in Hoopa Valley, California, about twenty-five miles east of Eureka, along the beautiful Trinity River. There was a Native American reservation there with a small, twenty-bed hospital, the Humboldt Medical Center; it seemed worth a drive to check it out.

I found a small but bright, clean hospital nestled in a small grove of stately redwood trees. Upon walking into the compact but well-equipped emergency room, I met with the hospital director to present my credentials and discuss the realities of rural and tribal medicine. I was offered a position to run the ER on a part-time basis. I accepted the position and felt that nothing could be more fitting, after all, for a young doctor who wanted to practice frontier medicine. Here I would be offering my services to descendants of those who had once lived vital, active lives in the North American forests before the white man came along to push forward the "frontier"—while, of course, thinning out its tree cover and, eventually, dotting it with fast-food chains.

Unfortunately, the physical condition of the patients to whom I attended on the reservation would have been something unrecognizable to their ancestors. A once-proud people had been reduced to a state that was sicker and even more obese and diabetic than the countless suburban Vancouver patients suffering from similar metabolic disorders whom I had so dearly desired to escape. Many Native Americans I treated suffered from alcoholism as well. Clearly, the white man's food and drink had done these folks no good at all. But I cared for them and tried to do the best I could for them.

Over time, I gradually gained the trust and friendship of some of my Native American patients, but there was always a pervasive sadness and a sense of futility to working there. As was the case with my patients in the Vancouver suburbs, the health of my Native American patients rarely improved despite my fervent pleas for them to swallow their medications, stab their fingers to check their blood sugars, and adjust their insulin dosages before eating. Again, I experienced far more success in treating their wounds than in dealing with their metabolic disorders. In addition, the grinding poverty and lack of opportunity, entertainment, and cultural offerings in the region gave a grimness to their lives—and to mine while trying to serve them. Three years of this work was enough.

Resigned to my failure as a general practitioner, whether in a big city or on the frontier, I decided to throw in the towel and become a specialist. I returned to Vancouver, where I had done a six-month traineeship program in anesthesiology in preparation for my foray into frontier medicine, now with the intention of completing my training in that field and becoming a board-certified anesthesiologist. I already had a six-month head start towards that certification, and, boy, that safe career path suddenly sounded good to me—not to mention lucrative.

It was during my residency in anesthesiology in 1981, while working in the cardiovascular unit of Vancouver General Hospital, that I got my first solid lesson on the primacy of diet to human health. A male heart patient who was scheduled for a heart bypass operation came in a couple of days earlier than usual before his scheduled surgery. The surgeons felt they needed more detailed angiograms, and the cardiologists wanted to do a day of heart monitoring, so the patient had a four-day inpatient stay before his scheduled surgery. Back in the 1970s and 1980s, Canadian hospitals often allowed stable patients scheduled for elective surgery to be given a day pass from the hospital to spend meaningful time with their families, as it might be the last time their families saw them relatively whole and functioning.

When that patient returned at the end of the day, the nurse noted that some required pre-op blood tests had not yet been done, and asked me if, while doing my rounds, I could please draw his blood. I did so and brought the blood samples up to the nurses' station, placing the tubes in a wire holding rack. After an hour or so attending to other patients in the ward, I came back to pick up the tubes, to take them down to the lab on my way to the OR. In the glass tubes, his blood had, of course, coagulated. The liquid part of the blood, the serum, floating above the dark red clot, is normally a crystal clear, transparent yellow. But this man's serum was a thick, milky white.

Now, I was aware of a condition called *postprandial lipemia* (fatty blood after eating). So, I knew that there could be fat in the blood after a meal. But this was the first time I had ever seen this stark phenomenon in the real world. I returned to the patient's bed and asked him if he had eaten while he was out with his family. He told me with delight that he had eaten his favorite meal: a double cheeseburger, French fries, and a milkshake. I realized then that what I had observed in the tubes were all the heavy fats the poor guy had just eaten: the beef fat in the burger, the egg yolk in the mayo on the bun, the butterfat in the cheese and milkshake, and the vegetable oil in the fried potatoes. It was all now flowing through his bloodstream. When held static in the blood tube, the food's fatty components showed their true colors and consistency. Upon analysis, the milky appearance of the serum was largely composed of triglycerides and saturated fats—the fats of the animals he had eaten.

Two days later, we took him to the OR, and I watched the surgeon open his chest and perform a coronary endarterectomy, a plaque-removing procedure that often precedes a coronary artery bypass graft. Delicately using forceps, the surgeon dissected out of the patient's coronary arteries a stiffer, fibrotic version of this same yellow slick that I had seen in the test tube—an almost perfect fatty cast of the blood-flow channel of his artery.

Although I hadn't actually witnessed the man eating the cheeseburgers that had contributed to his artery blockage, I felt like I had otherwise watched the entire process that is the etiology of heart disease play out before my eyes.

I was starting to comprehend that so much of what determines our health comes down, after all, to what we pour through our bloodstreams, day after day, month after month, year after year.

It takes the liver a good four or five hours, without eating, to begin to clear the fat eaten at a meal out of the bloodstream. During those four hours, damage is done to the blood vessel linings (the endothelium) and to most of the body's tissues by increasing inflammation and insulin resistance. Just when the liver is making progress in removing the disruptive fats and other molecular marauders from the bloodstream, guess what inevitably happens next? Answer: another fatty meal, usually containing another surge of animal-based foods (meat or dairy), often with a side of fried foods and a soda for extra helpings of free radicals.

I realized I was effectively watching people eat their way into life-threatening disease. Could I therefore help them eat their way out of it?

I had recently seen an article in a medical journal describing a case of a patient in the UK who had such severe angina pectoris that he had to stop every nine or ten paces.[2] He adopted a diet of whole plant foods and, within a half year, was hiking the mountains in the Lake District in England with no angina pain. From reading this and other studies, my left-brained, intellectual side was getting the message that adopting a diet of whole plant foods could apparently reverse atherosclerosis. I wondered if I needed to make that change myself, to avoid the same vascular catastrophes that were regularly befalling my medical patients.

A like message would soon be delivered to my right-brained, emotional, and moral side, in a most unexpected place.

In the second year of my three-year residency program, I had a fateful dinner at a local steakhouse. I dined there with a fellow anesthesiology resident named John, with whom I enjoyed having intellectual discussions. While polishing off a porterhouse steak, I found myself pontificating about living a life of nonviolence.

My friend didn't look particularly impressed. He cocked his head to one side and told me: "That's all very nice, Michael, but if you really want to get the violence out of your life, you might want to start with that piece of meat on your plate. Don't you see that as you satisfy your taste for flesh in your mouth, you are paying for the death of that animal, and for the next one in line at the slaughterhouse?"

And with that, John returned to eating his own steak, as if to make the point that he, at least, was no hypocrite, as he had never claimed to be a pacifist.

Several defensive rationales immediately flew through my mind: *"Well, the animal's dead already,"* or *"That's what they raise them for, after all,"* or *"Eating meat is all part of the circle of life."* But these defenses were so lame that I couldn't even bring myself to utter them. More persuasive than any of those rationalizations was the still, small voice in the back of my head telling me that John was right. Meat eating was, of course, thoroughly incompatible with pacifism. On my uncle's dairy farm, after all, I had seen more than enough old dairy cows shot in the head and butchered; that was inevitably their fate after their milk production declined to the point that they were no longer useful. (It is the dairy industry, after all, that enables the ground-beef industry—the source of the billions of burger patties served at fast-food outlets around the globe—while also inevitably generating the veal industry, which kills all male calves at four months.) I had chopped the heads off chickens and watched the life force drain from the severed hens' eyes. I knew the violence that was implicit in putting any animal foods on the plate. If I really wanted to shun violence in my life, I needed to start with my fork.

When I went to pay the bill for my steak dinner, I felt complicit in a crime. I loved those gentle bovine creatures and felt like their betrayer by savoring the taste of their flesh.

From that evening forward, I gave up red meat. Within a couple of weeks, I became explicitly and wholeheartedly vegan.

Learning of my new diet, a friend mentioned that he had recently visited a community of plant-based folks north of Orlando, Florida, in a place called Paisley. He suggested that I take a trip there to meet like-minded people. The idea sounded immediately appealing. I used my upcoming vacation time to go there, and it was an experience that proved life changing.

The community, which exists to this day (though it has relocated to Hawaii), was called Gentle World. It consisted of about thirty-five fit, healthy people in their twenties, thirties, and forties who lived in a communal environment and shared meals. And the food, much of it grown on their farm, was beyond wonderful. After years of eating meals based upon meats and dairy products, and frequent greasy, salty restaurant entrees, I now spent two weeks eating bowls of whole grains—brown rice, quinoa, and millet—with veggies and lentils or beans; satisfying stews, soups, chilies, and curries; a wide variety of colorful fruits, vital salads, plenty of leafy greens, fresh juices, and smoothies. I felt better than I had felt in years. After two weeks of eating more delicious, hearty meals than I could remember ever eating in my life, and quite possibly *more food* than I had ever eaten in my life, I discovered that I had lost eight pounds!

I returned to Vancouver to continue my anesthesiology residency, but my mind kept drifting back to those glorious two weeks of health and fitness, of warmth and kindness, and of energizing, living food in Florida. Within a few days of returning to the cardiovascular service, I spent a long day in the operating room, watching an obese cardiovascular surgeon perform a complex coronary bypass procedure and ventricular aneurism repair on an obese patient who had suffered a heart attack. When the long procedure was finally over, and the patient was verified to be still alive and stable, the surgical team headed straight down to the cafeteria to celebrate and refuel. There, I watched in amazement as that obese surgeon wolfed down a burger, a milkshake, and French fries.

I felt like I was working in a Fellini movie. Did nobody else in my field even suspect a relationship between food and health?

I could not deny to myself that my heart was no longer in this work. I didn't want to spend the rest of my life putting patients to sleep, when so many were suffering from conditions for which surgery was not the optimal answer. It was clear to me that the proper course was for my patients to change the way they lived and ate—and that I should do the same.

It was not truly a hard decision for me to walk away from my anesthesiology residency in Vancouver and a potentially lucrative career as a medical specialist. In my heart, I longed to return to the healthy community of plant-eating people in Florida where I had made so many new friends.

I left the anesthesia program and moved to Florida, finding work in an urgent care clinic outside of Orlando. In this high-flow clinic, as I cared for patients with metabolic disorders, if time allowed, after tending to the patient's acute need, I'd ask them what they were eating. If they were open to it, I'd give them a handout with suggestions for daily helpings of healthy, whole plant foods to eat for most or all of their meals.

Within weeks of starting to practice medicine in this new way, I received a phone call from a diabetic patient of mine who was complaining of headaches; his blood sugar level was way down in the forties.

"What have you been eating?" I asked him.

"I've been eating the way you told me to, doctor," he said. "I've lost fifteen pounds."

"Remind me how many units of insulin you're on?"

"Twelve units."

"Cut it to six units, and call me tomorrow."

He called the next day with essentially the same complaint, though his blood sugar had risen slightly; it was now in the fifties, but still dangerously low.

That's when I said those fateful words: "Stop your insulin, man. You don't have type 2 diabetes anymore."

As I spoke those words, I half expected to see a puff of smoke arise behind me and the ghost of my internal medicine professor appear, scowling and berating me: "Stopping a patient's insulin? Are you mad? Nobody gets off insulin!"

That's what we had been taught in medical school, in no uncertain terms. This was the first time I had ever given a medical order that explicitly contradicted the dogma that I had learned during my medical education. I felt a slight tinge of nervousness about doing so, but now I understood the mechanism by which this patient had reversed his diabetes: It was simply his diet, suddenly rich in whole plant foods and low in fat, that allowed his previously fat-clogged insulin receptors to open up and begin to function normally. As long as he continued to eat in such a low-fat, plant-based style, having him continue to inject insulin that he no longer needed would be irresponsible, even dangerous. Excess insulin would drop his blood sugar to perilously low levels, potentially causing damage to his brain and other organs. In this case, the "radical" order "Stop your insulin" was appropriate and necessary for me to issue and for the patient to hear.

He called me about ten days later to tell me that he was continuing to feel great and that his morning blood sugars were consistently below 116 mg/dL. I told him to follow up with his family doctor; he had already done so. Apparently, the family doctor was happy for him but never asked about what, exactly, the patient had done to reverse this serious chronic disease. (I would see this phenomenon reoccur for decades: The patient heals remarkably well through diet and reports that progress to a jaw-droppingly incurious physician.)

Shortly thereafter, another patient, who had been suffering from high blood pressure, also called me at the urgent care clinic. He, too, had followed my dietary instructions and had rapidly evolved his diet to one based upon whole plant foods. Now, having lost almost twenty pounds since I had first seen him in the clinic several weeks before, he was feeling very lightheaded when he stood up. He was concerned that he might pass out completely—not an unfounded fear, as the potent antihypertensive medications I had prescribed for him block the body's compensatory mechanisms of slight vasoconstriction and heart rate acceleration that keep blood flowing up to the brain, and they thus prevent us from passing out when we stand up. So the sensation that he felt as blood was draining from his head was real, and it truly did pose a threat that he would faint and, as he fell, strike his head or gash his face. Any such calamity would have been woefully iatrogenic—caused by the doctor and his ministrations. No wonder my heart sped up as I heard him report what he was experiencing.

I had him give me a home reading of his blood pressure while he was sitting quietly in a chair and then immediately after standing up; it was in the low-normal range on both readings, around 100/68 mm Hg. I told him to cut his blood pressure medication in half and call me in three days.

He called as promised and reported that even on half a dose of his medications, his blood pressure was still in the low-normal range, around 98/60 mm Hg, and he was concerned that he was still feeling lightheaded when he stood up. I congratulated him on apparently overcoming his hypertension, and I told him to eliminate his blood pressure medication entirely and to call me in three days.

Once again, I knew I had uttered a medical heresy. We were taught in medical school that once you put a patient on blood pressure medication, you must make it clear to them that it is a lifetime protocol of pills. After telling him to stop his medications, I glanced quickly behind me to again see if there was a puff of smoke swirling around the scowling ghost of my internal medicine professor, no doubt livid at my heretical advice. But, of course, there was no puff of smoke, and I wasn't struck by lightning. I must admit that it felt a little odd at first to take a patient off his blood pressure medication, but I understood that it was only because, for the first time in my career, I was actually helping patients with metabolic disorders to reverse their diseases.

I told the patient to follow up with his family doctor, which he did. He later wrote me that his doctor was pleased with his progress but not at all curious about how he had accomplished this remarkable medical turnaround. Sound familiar?

Gradually, and increasingly, this became my way of practicing medicine. When the opportunity allowed, I spoke with patients about their diet, and I advised them to follow a plant-predominant diet—as close to a low-fat, whole-food, plant-exclusive diet as I felt I could persuade them to go. I explained to them the basis for that request and how it related to their disease state. I gave them handouts to suggest foods that they should and should not eat. I followed up with them, when I could, about their dietary progress. When they were able to follow the dietary instructions I gave, I repeatedly found that they were able to improve or even totally overcome their metabolic disorders such as high blood pressure and type 2 diabetes, and thus they were able to significantly reduce or even stop their medications altogether.

With newfound clarity, I realized that *Etiology Unknown* was not, as I had once generously believed, a humble expression of the current limitations of scientific knowledge. Nor was it a statement of the mysterious nature of our leading killers. There is in fact little that is mysterious about the causes of heart disease, hypertension, type 2 diabetes, obesity, and a raft of other diseases rampant in our country. Almost always, these diseases are brought on by the extraordinarily fatty Western diet, built around animal foods and processed foods full of refined sugars and oils. These effects are only exacerbated by a high-stress, sedentary lifestyle.

Etiology Unknown was nothing more than willful blindness. The yellow gunk clogging the arteries of Americans, and of people who eat the Western diet all over the world, is the predictable result of that fatty, sweet diet of animal foods, sugars, and oils.

Etiology Unknown, intended to be a scientific-sounding characterization of a mystery, has in fact one thing truly mysterious about it: why educated men and women, presumably dedicated to a healing profession, would want to either fool themselves or to convince others that what is known and blatantly obvious is unknown.

Etiology Unknown, my gluteus.

Chapter Two

THE TOXIC RED TIDE

Let us begin with an understanding of a fact that should be obvious: A healthy bloodstream is vital to our well-being.

After eating any meal, every molecule absorbed from your food flows through your bloodstream and becomes involved in an ongoing exchange with the molecules composing your heart, your lungs, your liver, your kidneys, your brain—in fact, all your organs.

It would therefore take an extraordinary act of faith to believe that the physical quality and composition of the blood circulating throughout the body, perfusing every living cell, do not directly affect one's health. Nonetheless, much of the medical establishment appears to hold to that faith. It is with no small amount of embarrassment and wonder that I report to you that it is the ingrained tendency of Western medicine, from its medical schools to its neighborhood clinics, to all but ignore the nature and composition of the blood coursing through our arteries. That is Western medicine's consistent approach when it formulates protocols to address disease, creates nutritional guidelines for our citizenry, and develops the next generation of medicines and surgical procedures. Judging by the public pronouncements of our leading medical authorities, the curricula of our medical schools, and the protocols of most conventional Western doctors in treating metabolic conditions, it doesn't appear to matter at all to our medical establishment whether your blood is fatty and viscous as light cream, with diminished capacity to deliver nutrients to your cells, or clear, free-flowing, and healthy. It's an afterthought, at best.

Knowing what we now know about how food affects our bodies and how it gets metabolized within us, this disinterest in blood quality, composition, and function represents an approach to health that falls somewhere between madness and malpractice.

The Physical Consequences of Our Food Stream

The majority of the patients I have attended to as a physician in a career now entering its second half century have suffered from the self-inflicted wound of the "Toxic Red Tide": repeatedly flooding their bloodstream with surges of damaging fats; oxidizing sugars; free-radical-laden fried foods; emulsifying agents; an array of flavorings, colorings, and additives; and a host of other disruptive chemical agents inherent in a daily diet laden with meats, dairy products, ubiquitous sugars and oils, and processed foods. Over time, with every meal composed of these elements—whether fast food, prepared at home, or served at a three-star Michelin restaurant—these lethal legions inflict molecular chaos in enzyme systems and cells throughout the body. The accumulated cellular damage initiates, and then fuels, the disease processes we physicians spend most of our careers treating.

The repeated infliction of fatty, animal-based meals and sugary, processed foods into the human body means that the fats and other disrupting molecules rarely clear out of the bloodstream. When you keep your blood fatty and sugary for twenty, thirty, or forty years, you shouldn't be shocked when some abnormal changes show up in your body.

Let's consider some of the physiologic consequences of such a food stream. First, there is the matter of blood viscosity: Think of it as the relative ease of flow of the stream of blood cells and plasma constituents that pour through vital but tiny capillary beds supplying the brain, heart, and other vital organs. For hours after a fatty meal, the fat coats the red cells, making it easier for them to stick to each other, resulting in a thicker blood flow that requires a higher blood pressure to force the blood through those tiny capillaries. Since most people on the Western diet are keeping their blood fatty pretty much all day, the constant high pressure required from the heart pump can eventually damage the heart muscle fibers, leading to congestive heart failure.

As the fat that is almost constantly in the omnivore's bloodstream infiltrates the muscle cells (then earning the label "intramyocellular lipid"), it inhibits enzymes in the insulin receptors on the surface of those cells. The insulin is then unable to perform its essential function of escorting glucose into the cell to be burned for energy. This increases insulin resistance and contributes to hours of high blood sugar levels.

The fat also infiltrates liver cells in a way that makes them insensitive to insulin's message to stop glycogenolysis—the conversion of glycogen stored in the liver and muscle cells to glucose. With the liver's insulin receptors clogged with fat, glycogenolysis continues unchecked, and the liver cells continue to pour sugar into the bloodstream. As sugar builds up in the bloodstream, it creates the hallmark elevated glucose levels that afflict those with diabetes (and somewhat less elevated levels of those with prediabetes). Unfortunately, these folks (along with those who merely fear diabetes) often then make the dietary choice to combat (or prevent) high blood sugar levels by avoiding those bad "carbs," not realizing that the high blood sugars are the effect, not the cause, of the insulin resistance. The real culprits are the dietary fats in the meats, dairy products, oils, and processed junk foods. Refined carbohydrates (sugars) in flours, sweets, and sodas certainly exacerbate the problem of high blood sugar. But the naturally occurring carbohydrates in the fiber, starches, and sugars of whole fruits, vegetables, and whole grains do not present a problem, and these foods should not be restricted.

What are the other, likely effects of keeping one's bloodstream fatty and sugary over time?

You may become overweight (with a BMI of between 25 kg/m2 and 30 kg/m2) or obese (with a BMI of over 30 kg/m2), both states that raise your risk of developing cancer of the colon, breast, or prostate.

You may develop high blood pressure, which elevates your risk of a stroke or heart attack or congestive heart failure.

You may experience chest tightness and difficulty walking up a flight of stairs—the condition called *angina pectoris*, which is a manifestation of often-lethal coronary artery disease.

All of these diseases have less to do with our genes and far more to do with our diet. We label them and treat them as the distinct conditions that they are, while ignoring the reality that they are all fundamentally related: They are the body's varied reactions to an unnatural stream of food being processed by a nutritionally stressed body and carried to your organs by an often-compromised bloodstream.

As unpleasant as it may be to contemplate, after every meal loaded with meat, dairy, sugar, and salt, there is an evil brew of molecules flowing through your blood for hours. What, exactly, are the problematic substances in the fatty Western diet? Sadly, the list is long, and it includes: excessive sodium and sugars, advanced glycation end products (AGEs), oxidized cholesterol, reactive aldehydes, Neu5Gc (N-glycolylneuraminic acid), insulin-like growth factor-1 (IGF-1), endotoxin, trimethylamine N-oxide (TMAO), carcinogenic heterocyclic amines, heme iron, emulsifiers, animal tissue peptides, free radicals in fried foods, bio-concentrated pesticides, herbicides, heavy metals, hormones, antibiotics, and microplastics.

Salt

Let's start with salt, a pitfall in the diets of meat eaters, vegetarians, and vegans alike. In the West, we generally consume a high-sodium diet. Of course, we humans all need some sodium in our diet, but we can get all we need from whole plant foods, which absorb sodium from the soil.

Unfortunately, too many people spend their days consuming extraordinarily salty foods like cheese (a substance that is unpalatable without salt), chips, fries, and many processed foods.

What's the problem with too much salt? Well, chemically, salt is a crystal of sodium and chloride atoms held together by their electric charges, and when the crystal dissolves in water (or in the bloodstream), the sodium atoms disassociate from the chloride and then infiltrate the walls of the arteries and stiffen them. The artery walls then lose the lovely elasticity that absorbs the shock waves from the heart's powerful ventricular contractions. And at the same time, in response to the salt surge in the blood, the kidneys retain water they would normally excrete in the urine in order to dilute the salt. This increases the total amount of blood in the circulatory system (the "intravascular volume") from, say, five liters to over six liters. As a result of both stiffer arteries and increased intravascular volume, blood pressure usually goes up.

In addition, we're finding out that sodium is not benign on an immunological level. High-salt diets stimulate the Th17 lymphocytes; this can open the door to autoimmune diseases such as lupus and painful inflammatory conditions such as ankylosing spondylitis.

Sugar

Then there's sugar. Used as an occasional flavoring, minute amounts of refined sugar may be relatively harmless. But when consumed in far greater amounts in baked goods, candies, and soft drinks—in addition to being hidden in all kinds of highly processed foods, from white bread to ketchup—sugar becomes dangerous. When you eat cakes and cookies, consider that you are in reality eating—let's face it—a chunk of sugar held together by some kind of fat (butter, egg yolk, shortening). With every bite of the treat, many grams of fructose, maltose, dextrose, and other sugars flood through your tissues. The sugars stick to proteins all over your body, such as the collagen in your connective tissue and the hemoglobin in your blood—a process known as *glycosylation*.

The human body didn't evolve to handle the mixing of sugars and proteins to this degree and intensity. As the sugar overload proceeds, strands of structural collagen and elastin proteins in skin—fibrils that should move independently like cables to support the skin's youthful structure—now stick to parts of their neighboring collagen strands, a process called *cross-linking*. Protein fibers in the dermis layer mat together into thick, gummed-up sheets that, with movement of the hands, arms, and face, buckle, crease, and eventually tear, producing the appearance of cracked, aged skin.

Enzymes are proteins within cells that are meant to be supple and able to wrap around and attach to binding sites of various molecules and cellular structures, where they catalyze chemical reactions and then lightly let go. But, when glycosylated with syrupy simple sugars, enzyme proteins distort, fold abnormally, and stick to parts of themselves or neighbors—another form of cross-linking—rendering themselves chemically useless.

Simple Sugars Cause Cross-Linking of Enzymes

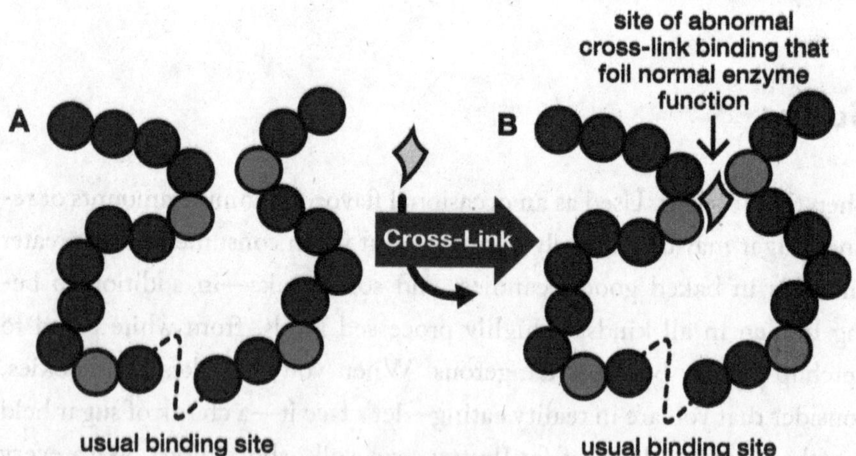

Flooding cell enzymes and structural proteins with sugar molecules can cause a protein chain to stick to itself, changing its shape and interfering with its function.

Further damage from the sugar-protein mash-up occurs when our body heat of 98.6°F (37°C) oxidizes the glycosylated sugar, a piece of chemistry called the *Maillard reaction*, a phenomenon with which every baker is familiar (whether they know the name for it or not). When baking, the sugar in pastry flour combines with, and glycosylates, the protein in wheat gluten, and the glycosylated protein is exposed to the oven's heat. The result is a mass of oxidized sugars and proteins called *advanced glycation end products*, whose battalions teem with free radicals—atoms missing an electron. In the body, the AGE molecules efficiently rip electrons off any nearby molecule, including from your cell membranes, plasma proteins, cholesterol, or DNA.

The Maillard reaction is a baker's boon in the oven but a bane in your body. The AGEs that form on the surface of a loaf of bread dough in the oven are prized as fragrant crust, which may be fine on the surface of a French baguette. But you don't want to run the Maillard reaction in the crystalline proteins of the lens of your eye; that is an invitation to form cataracts, as the lens proteins fracture and block the passage of light on its way to the retina. You don't want to run the Maillard reaction in the endothelium of the blood vessels in your brain; that would inhibit the flow of oxygen and nutrients needed to nourish your neurons. This silent sabotage goes on after each meal of fried foods and baked goods. It's a good reason to remember the acronym: AGEs. Eating sugar as a food AGEs you.

Eating Animal Muscle

As you can see, merely avoiding animal foods does not ensure that your bloodstream won't carry inflammatory toxins to your tissues. A slice of vegan cheesecake can be as fatty, salty, and sugary as a slice of traditional cheesecake and do significant harm. Junk food—food-like substances that are heavy with salt, sugar, and/or fat, designed to maximize taste pleasure while being devoid of useful nutrients—vegan or not, should be absolutely minimized or, better, avoided entirely.

Still, for most Americans, it's the animal foods that do the most damage.

What happens when we eat what we call "meat," which is truly just a euphemism for animal muscle? Well, start with the reality that almost nobody eats raw animal muscle, after all. It's usually cooked—fried, roasted, grilled, or baked. And remember a biologic fact: Every animal muscle cell contains cholesterol. Over the hot flame, in the oven, on the grill, the cholesterol gets oxidized—that is, loses an electron.

Every time you eat cooked meat, you're sending a flood of oxidized cholesterol particles through your bloodstream. Oxidized cholesterol does you no good, promoting atherosclerotic plaque formation and inflammation. It crosses the blood-brain barrier and has been found in Alzheimer's plaques.

The very act of broiling a steak, frying a chicken, or grilling a fish oxidizes not only cholesterol but also nucleic acids and proteins in the animal's muscle. This toxic chemistry consequently creates a whole slew of reactive aldehydes, with names like malondialdehyde, glyoxal dialdehyde, and acrolein. These are nasty molecules, small but chemically vicious, as they are mutagenic; that is, they damage your DNA strands, the genes that they contain, and the essential cellular enzymes they produce. You surely don't want to damage your genes with a bunch of reactive aldehydes just because there's a convenient fast-food joint close by for lunch, but every cooked burger and chicken breast and buffalo wing sends a flood of those nefarious agents through your bloodstream, each on a sabotage mission to damage your cells.

Then there's good old Neu5Gc (N-Glycolylneuraminic acid). You probably haven't heard of this compound. I hadn't myself, until a few years ago. It's a sialic acid (a synthesized sugar) that other mammals synthesize, but humans cannot. In the human body, it's highly inflammatory, and there's reason for concern that it may pose carcinogenic risk.[1] If you use special stains and search for it under a microscope, you can find Neu5Gc in the coronary artery lesions and in the membranes of rheumatoid arthritic joints. Thus, it's a suspected contributor to atherosclerotic disease, rheumatoid arthritis, and other conditions now known to be driven by inflammation. I'm afraid that our meat-advocating Paleo diet enthusiasts are giving themselves a shot of Neu5Gc with every flesh-based meal.

When you eat a piece of meat, prized for its protein content, a barrage of amino acids floods into the liver. That organ responds by producing a surge of insulin-like growth factor-1 (IGF-1), one of the most powerful growth-promoting hormones in the body. IGF-1 serves the important purpose of driving cell proliferation when you're a growing child, but if you're an adult woman with an early-stage breast cancer, or if you're a man with an enlarged prostate and some malignant cells inside of it, the last thing you want is a diet that makes you walk around with cell-proliferating IGF-1 in your blood. Unfortunately, that's exactly what a diet of flesh foods and dairy foods (made from milk sufficiently rich in IGF-1 to enable a baby calf to grow into a four-hundred-pound cow in six to ten months) creates. The Standard American Diet predictably produces unhealthy blood levels of IGF-1 and other growth hormones that may drive cancer growth in the tissues of the breast, prostate, and other organs.[2]

The meat-based diet also mounts a bodily assault by endotoxins. Doctors understand how harmful such an assault can be, as those who spend time in the intensive care unit often encounter a dreadful, widely feared phenomenon called *endotoxic shock*; this occurs when a storm of bacteria in the gut escapes into the bloodstream and releases a family of small, lethal molecules called *endotoxins*. The resulting condition of endotoxemia shuts down organs; causes excessive, uncontrolled inflammation and vasodilation (widening of the blood vessels), which may disseminate blood clotting; and even, in extreme circumstances, may cause death.

Where does dietary endotoxin come from? Its origin is in the slaughterhouse. Virtually every animal that gets eaten passes through the slaughterhouse—yes, even organic, grass-fed beef; "regeneratively raised" meat; halal and kosher meat. After the animal has its throat severed and is hung up on the rack, it is eviscerated. And when the GI system is removed from the carcass, the gut bacteria (kosher or not) naturally spill out. As a result, you can take a culture tube from the microbiology lab and swipe most every cutting surface in the slaughterhouse and find teeming populations of *Salmonella*, *E. coli*, *Shigella*, *Pseudomonas*, *Enterococcus*—the whole rogues' gallery of disease-producing enteric bacteria. Expect no fewer of these disease-producing strains of bacteria from the organic, regenerative, halal, and kosher-killed cows as from the "conventional" cows. That means that every steak, every lamb chop, and every chicken breast that has encountered this cutting surface has a film of enteric bacteria on its surface.

The flesh food is then wrapped in clear, plastic wrap and sent to the supermarket. There it sits in the meat case under an ultraviolet light that shines down to kill the bacteria. As a result of the ultraviolet light, and certainly of cooking at sufficient temperatures, these bacteria die. Unfortunately, when they do, their cell walls break apart, releasing endotoxins.

You want to know what endotoxins do? Take a look at the "Daisy of Death."

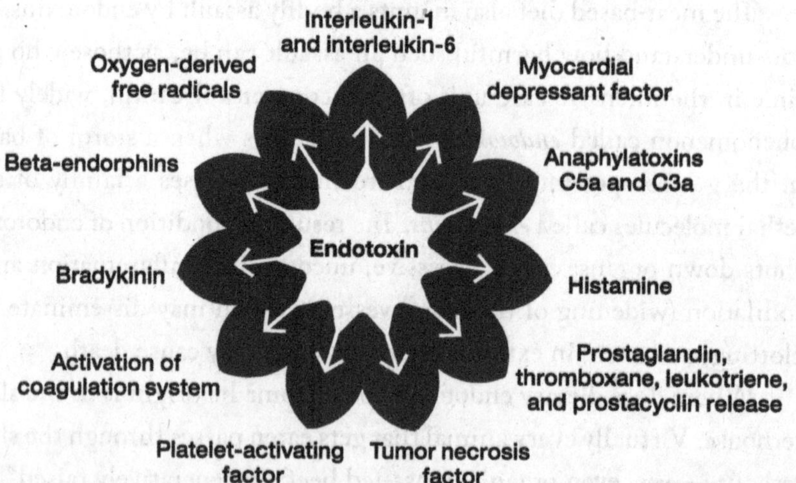

The Daisy of Death: toxic substances whose release is triggered by endotoxins.

In this image, you see the myriad effects of endotoxins on our bodies. They release surges of inflammation-inciting free radicals (damaging DNA), depress the myocardium (causing dysfunction of both sides of the heart), release histamine (making capillaries leaky), release tumor necrosis factor (TNF, which plays a role in the development of cancers), activate the coagulation system (setting off blood clotting), and release pro-inflammatory prostaglandin E2 and interleukin-1 and 6 (all contributing to autoimmune and inflammatory conditions) and thromboxane (which can further fuel blood clots), as well as anaphylatoxins (peptides that stoke inflammation).

Making all these risks worse, the absorption of endotoxins is enhanced by fat in the diet.[3] That's a remarkably inconvenient fact, since the very foods that are introducing the endotoxins into the bloodstream—burgers and fried chicken, for example—are by nature high-fat foods.

Even worse still, endotoxins are heat stable. Cooking the burger or grilling the chicken does not get rid of the endotoxins; they survive the cooking only to inflict their cellular damage, first in the wall of the intestine and then in distant tissues as they escape into the bloodstream. With their flesh-based meals, our keto and Paleo diet friends give themselves a shot of endotoxins two or three times a day. I fear that they're going to find out the hard way that endotoxins make your gut leaky, as these molecules increase intestinal permeability. That allows food proteins and the cell walls of bacteria to leak into the bloodstream and flow through important tissues throughout the body, including joint membranes, opening the door to inflammatory arthritis and autoimmune diseases. These diseases take years to appear, but adherents to flesh-based diets would seem to be inviting these afflictions.

The grim parade of toxins from a meat-besotted diet continues with TMAO. What is that? Well, we have by now learned a central lesson concerning the microbiome in our intestines: The food you eat determines the microbes that thrive in your gut. If you eat a lot of sugar, for example, you're going to summon up a wave of sugar-eating microbes. Eat a diet based on meat and eggs, and you'll be dropping a steady stream of carnitine and choline down into your gut, fostering a vigorous population of microbes that thrive by metabolizing carnitine and choline. They have names like *Peptostreptococcaceae* and *Clostridiaceae*, and although these microbes live rent free inside you, they are the most ungrateful of tenants. They don't care about you; they're waiting for that next chicken breast or salmon steak to come down the pipe, and they will metabolize the carnitine and choline into trimethylamine, which your liver then promptly oxidizes into trimethylamine N-oxide, or TMAO.

And TMAO is a molecule from hell. It drives cholesterol into the artery walls and interferes with HDL's role in accomplishing reverse transport (removal) of cholesterol from the artery walls. TMAO is implicated in the development of both heart disease and kidney disease.[4] One published study has already shown that long-term Paleo eaters have significantly elevated TMAO concentrations,[5] putting them at higher risk for often lethal cardiac events.

Cooking animal muscle at high temperatures inevitably creates a family of cancer-causing heterocyclic amines; these multi-ring molecules set off malignancies in many tissues that they contact, including the stomach wall. Meat-based eaters suffer a much higher incidence of gastric cancers than do vegetarians.[6]

Of special interest to all owners of a colon, the fecal matter of meat eaters is replete with carcinogens. As a 2015 study published in *Oncology Review* reported: "NOCs [N-nitroso compounds] are mutagenic and potent carcinogenic agents in animals . . . NOCs can be formed also endogenously after consumption of red and processed meat. . . . Total N-nitroso compounds in fecal samples were found increased after high red meat intake in volunteers."[7] As there's no fiber in meat, the fecal mass moves through the colon slowly, providing a long exposure time for these carcinogenic molecules to smear against the descending colon wall. Therefore, it's no surprise that meat eaters develop far more carcinomas of the descending and sigmoid colon than do vegetarians.[8]

Then there's heme iron—the iron attached to animal hemoglobin, which we absorb when we ingest flesh foods. Iron in small amounts plays the crucial role of allowing your bone marrow to generate hemoglobin, the vital pigment that permits red blood cells to ferry oxygen to all the body's tissues. But an excess of iron should be avoided. Just look at a rusty car bumper and you're reminded that iron is a pro-oxidant that catalyzes chemical damage in most of the molecules it encounters. It does not spare the molecules of proteins in cell membranes or even the precious DNA in the very nucleus of the cells.

When you've got iron overload in your body, you're at higher risk for strokes and GI cancers as well. In fact, a 2018 study found that "Increased intracellular iron . . . has diverse roles in the initiation, growth, and metastasis of cancer cells."[9] So, the avid red meat eater may be helping early cancers avidly spread to distant parts of their body.

While we all need iron, we can relax knowing that there's plenty of iron in plant foods—in dark leafy greens, in pumpkin seeds, in all legumes, and in dried fruits, such as raisins, prunes, and apricots. Consequently, as with sodium, you get all the iron you need from a varied diet of plant foods that absorb the mineral from the ground.

Now, the iron in plants is not heme iron, and that's a good thing, as your intestinal lining can effectively regulate the amount of non-heme iron that it allows to be absorbed into your bloodstream. If the iron stores in your bone marrow are full, your gut wall can keep out non-heme iron, thus protecting you from the perils of iron overload. But your gut has no such control over heme iron, which just leaps into the bloodstream full throttle. Men who eat steak after steak risk giving themselves iron overload because we males, as well as postmenopausal women, cannot easily rid ourselves of excess iron.

Iron overload may also lead to greater susceptibility to infection; another 2018 study found that "Iron is an essential nutrient for bacterial survival and thus higher iron levels may precipitate bacterial infections."[10]

These days, the Toxic Red Tide commonly carries emulsifiers used by the food industry for such purposes as keeping ice cream soft and creamy. But these emulsifiers can do more than that. They can also dissolve the mucus layer protecting our intestinal lining, thus allowing fragments of animal muscle protein and cell walls of dead bacteria to pass into the bloodstream, setting off inflammation and possible autoimmune disease.

Finally, there are the synthetic, human-created toxins in meat. Feedlot animals are fed bushels of grains that have been sprayed with pesticides and herbicides. These pesticides and herbicides then bio-accumulate in the animals' flesh. What makes that chicken so finger-lickin' good to those addicted to the Western diet is the fat in the muscles of those birds. And the fat is where these toxins accumulate, as they are fat-soluble substances. Let's not forget, either, that the water in the feedlot is never filtered or distilled. So it's often going to contain heavy metals like mercury and cadmium that, of course, wind up in that animal flesh as well.

Recognizing the flood of disruptive molecules that pour through your tissues in the wake of eating animal foods, it's hard to imagine how any burger, lamb chop, steak, or chicken breast can be considered safe or proper nourishment for human beings.

Of course, most people have not been informed of these facts. While meat eaters often discover the risks of their diet the hard way—when they receive some daunting diagnosis, or fall victim to a heart attack or stroke—they are usually then shielded from the knowledge that their animal-based diet likely played a major role in bringing on their disease. They are told that they simply have bad genes—or bad luck.

Eating Fish

"Well, I don't eat meat; I just eat fish." You hear that line of defense a lot. Unfortunately, a meal of fish is also a meal of muscle that shares much in common with the muscles of mammals. But fish present a special danger of their own: We've been treating the oceans like sewers, so most of our large game fish are replete with mercury, pesticides, dioxins, and, now, microplastics. Fish flesh now inevitably contains innumerable tiny shards of polyethylene and other plastics, much of it from the decomposing plastic bags, trash, and discarded fishnets that float on our oceans in huge patches known as *gyres*, some twice the size of Texas. Since much of the world's fish catch is ground up and added to animal feed for billions of chickens, cows, and pigs, the ocean load of microplastics works its way up to the omnivore's dinner plate on a daily basis. It is estimated that meat-eating Americans now ingest a credit card's (five grams) worth of microplastics every week from the food they eat and water they drink![11] Since the body has no enzymes to break down or eliminate these plastics, they accumulate in our tissues with yet unknown effects—but one can assume they will not be positive ones. In chapter 4 we will discuss the link between seafood and neurological diseases.

Farmed fish present essentially the same class of dangers as those posed by land animals in concentrated feeding operations: Crowded together in unnatural conditions, large, predator fish such as salmon swim around in their own waste. They are fed or injected with antibiotics in a dubious effort to prevent fungal and parasitic infections but are often afflicted with open sores nonetheless. As a further worry, farmed salmon often contain high concentrations of such chemical poisons as polychlorinated biphenyls (PCBs).

Wild-caught fish present a different danger: Many are infested with parasites that the consumer may not see. Wild fish, after all, eat the eggs of parasites in the water; that's not a behavior that humans can arrest. One Danish study found that "Parasitic nematodes of the family Anisakidae [roundworms] occur in the visceral cavity and surrounding tissues of many marine fish species at a prevalence as high as 100 percent in wild salmon samples. Human consumption of fish products containing these parasites can result in the zoonotic disease anisakiasis, and Anisakis simplex is most commonly associated with human disease."[12] That same study found that the risk of parasites in fish was 570 times worse in wild salmon than farmed salmon. Humans who eat undercooked fish also run the risk of acquiring fish tapeworms (*Diphyllobothrium latum*) that can grow to over twenty feet long inside the human body. So if you're a fish eater, pick your poison: antibiotics and PCBs in farmed fish, parasites in wild-caught fish, and mercury, dioxin, and microplastics across the board. Of course, it's hard to know where your fish is coming from, anyway, as the labeling you encounter in the market might not be trustworthy.

A Lifetime of Toxins

For doctors, understanding the Red Tide that surges through our tissues with every meal of animal-based foods requires us to focus a very sharp lens on our patients' diets and adds life-or-death significance to the nutritional advice that we dispense. It presents this question to the clinician: Does your patient's blood carry these molecules meal after meal, day after day, perfusing every tissue in their body, or does it not? Because if physicians acquiesce to the standard Western diet, or, even worse, if they promote a carnivore or keto diet, they are in effect telling the patient: "Animal foods and their abundant fats are good for you; I want you to keep these menacing molecules percolating through every tissue in your body—your brain, your heart, your kidneys, your bone marrow—meal after meal, hour after hour, day after day, week after week, month after month. Just keep an abundant supply of these nutritional saboteurs in your viscous, rich bloodstream pretty much constantly, and then come back to me if you develop any symptoms that concern you."

I will remind the reader that the Colorado River carved the Grand Canyon one minute, one hour, one day at a time, year after year . . . this is the power of persistence. And yet we doctors have effectively been telling our patients: *Yup, keep these molecules flowing through your bloodstream and your tissues, pretty much constantly over the course of your lifetime.* We shouldn't then act surprised when tissues become inflamed in the body or when the arteries start clogging with plaque. We shouldn't be mystified that the gut has gotten leaky, nor then be puzzled about where that lupus came from. We shouldn't attribute colon cancer to unlucky genetics or pretend that the causes of our most common diseases are unknown.

We practice medicine as if what our patients eat has no effect on these diseases. As scientists, how can we do so with a straight face? How can we ignore this very powerful disruptive influence to which our patients subject themselves daily—usually with our silent acquiescence stemming from a disinterest in nutrition, and occasionally even with our blessing and encouragement?

I say to my medical colleagues: *When your patients sit in front of you—overweight or obese, atherosclerotic, hypertensive, diabetic, and inflamed—do you ask them what they have been eating? Is your patient pouring these deleterious substances through their bloodstream, meal after meal? If so, they need your honest counsel to set them on the nutritional path that will lead them away from disease and towards vibrant health.*

The WPF Diet

We know that the whole plant food diet will immediately and effectively staunch this onslaught of these very toxic molecules. My question to my fellow physicians then is: "Do you inform your patients of that fact?" If you do not, you do your patients a disservice by merely dispensing medicines to treat their symptoms while ignoring the underlying causation of their diseases.

Let me pause now to define what I mean by a whole plant food (WPF) diet, as the term will be used throughout this book. Do I mean simply a vegan diet? Of course not. A vegan diet could be a diet of vegan donuts, potato chips, and beer. "Vegan" simply defines what one is *not* eating (animal products); it says nothing about what one *is* eating.

The term "whole food plant-based" (WFPB) has often been used as an alternative to "vegan" for just that reason: to make clear that one's diet should optimally be centered on whole foods—plant foods eaten more or less as grown, rather than processed. A WFPB diet has the benefit of excluding, say, vegan cupcakes. My objection to using the term "whole food plant-based" is that I do not know how to define "plant-based." The term is vague enough that some people might apply it to their diet even if they eat red meat and/or chicken and/or fish and/or eggs and/or dairy once or twice every week, or maybe even once or twice a day, as long as they satisfy themselves that they are consuming the bulk of their calories from plants. I could never endorse such a diet, even while I would grant that it's less injurious to one's health than a diet commanding the bulk of its calories from animal foods.

A whole plant food diet, by contrast, is indeed a vegan (not just vaguely "plant-based") diet centered on unprocessed or minimally processed whole plant foods: vegetables (including sea vegetables), fruits, whole grains, mushrooms (which are technically not plants but rather fungi), legumes, nuts, and seeds.

Most of the foods eaten on a whole plant food diet will be found in the produce section of the grocery store, but others can be found in the bulk bins or as packaged foods (nuts, seeds, grains, legumes, and seaweed). But there are also some foods—let's call them the "exception foods"—that may not jump to mind as perfect examples of "whole plant foods," yet I would include them as acceptable foods that can add variety to a WPF diet, while making it easier to adopt. These "exception foods" include whole grain, vegan breads, as well as tortillas, pastas, ramen noodles, and polenta; the soy-based staples of tofu and tempeh; nondairy, unsweetened yogurts; oil-free, sugar-free plant milks; nutritional yeast; refined sugar-free jams; and dried fruits.

Let's break these down further to prevent a slide into a diet of unhealthy, processed foods.

Breads, again, should be made from whole grains, which means, for example, that the ingredients should list "whole wheat" rather than simply "wheat." Look for breads with a minimal list of ingredients. Breads made from sprouted grains, such as the Ezekiel breads, will be the healthiest.

The same whole grain preference applies to **pastas** as well, but there are also acceptable pastas made from such diverse ingredients as legume flours and Jerusalem artichoke flour. Even regular semolina pasta will not hurt you, as long as you are not gluten sensitive.

Tofu and tempeh are staple foods in many WPF diets that provide very ample quantities of protein; I'm including them with the "exception foods" only in that they are somewhat processed foods—but not processed in a way that will be deleterious to your health. In fact, tofu and tempeh are health promoting; just make sure you do not eat them fried.

Brown, black, red, and purple rice are preferable to white rice, but once in a while, especially if you're in a restaurant in which you have no other choice, white rice is acceptable.

Choose a **nondairy yogurt** that is made without any oil (pro-inflammatory, artery-clogging coconut oil has become ubiquitous in the "natural food" industry and should be assiduously avoided) and that is unsweetened; you can sweeten it yourself, if you wish, with fruit-sweetened jam.

Plant milks made from nuts, hemp seeds, oats, or soy are all acceptable, but make sure they are made without oil and are unsweetened.

Jams should be sweetened only with fruit or fruit concentrate, not with refined sugar.

Dried fruits should be consumed sparingly, as their sugar concentration can be very high.

While the guidelines I'm providing here for what constitutes a WPF diet may be too liberal for some purists, and perhaps too strict for some processed-food enthusiasts, I think they are realistic. I don't believe that the occasional breakfast of, say, whole grain sprouted bread with pure all-fruit organic blueberry jam will hurt you; indeed, it will be far healthier than most breakfasts that Americans eat. Still, don't over-rely on these somewhat processed "exception foods"; instead, base your WPF diet on the foods that you will find in the produce section of your grocery store or in the bulk bins: whole fruits and vegetables, whole grains, and legumes, plus a sprinkling of nuts and seeds. Make sure to eat your leafy greens at least once a day—more, if possible—and experiment to find the right percentage of calories from raw fruits and vegetables that works for you.

For most people, a diet that is composed of at least 20 percent (by calorie) raw fruits and vegetables works well. For some sugar-sensitive people (and for those suffering from fatty liver disease), too many fruits (contributing too much fructose) may pose a problem, and those people may need to limit fruits to, say, two or three servings per day. They may find as well that they fare better when consuming low-fructose fruits such as berries, kiwi, and cantaloupe, as opposed to high-fructose fruits such as ripe bananas, grapes, mangoes, and pears—but all of these are healthy foods, notwithstanding.

Creating your own optimal WPF diet may seem daunting at first and may take some time to perfect. You have to factor in practicalities like how much time and energy you can devote to preparing meals, your taste preferences, how you feel after eating certain foods, and which foods may trigger overeating (breads, pastas, nuts, and dried fruit come to mind). You might also want to challenge yourself to experiment by tasting whole plant foods that are new to you. By monitoring your bloodwork, you may be able to divine how certain foods and dietary patterns affect your health metrics.

If you suffer from virtually any metabolic condition, the WPF diet is the necessary first step, and sometimes the only step, that you need to take to reverse your condition. If you need to lose weight, strict adherence to the WPF diet will gradually bring you to your optimal weight. Minimization of the fattiest foods permitted on the WPF diet (nuts, seeds, avocado, tofu, olives, coconut) and the most calorically dense nonfatty foods (bread, tortillas, dried fruit) will facilitate weight loss. Your weight loss on a WPF diet will be achieved in a manner consistent with your health, which is its great advantage when compared to other diets, such as the Paleo diet or keto diet, which may sometimes result in short-term weight loss, but only at the expense of your long-term health.

Drive-By Nutritional Advice

Paleo enthusiasts, convinced by fad diet books that humans should eat the way Paleo-promoting authors imagine cavemen ate, seem hell-bent on risking their health for short-term weight loss and apparent improvement in some lab test numbers, like HgbA1c. When people adopt these diets, they often improve initially. "*Oh, my, I went on a Paleo diet and lost weight, and my blood sugars got better; I feel great.*" I grant that happens. One reason that happens is that dairy is not part of the Paleo diet; as presumably no caveman ever milked a cow, the Paleo advocates disapprove of dairy, and good for them on that point. No caveman ever squeezed the fat out of olives and poured it on their salad, so they're down on oil, and they're right. No caveman ever pounded wheat into flour and made donuts and coffee cakes, so they're down on pastries, and again they're right. When you eliminate the dairy and the oils and the flours from your diet, you are likely going to trim down some, especially if you have a lot of weight to lose. The weight loss will provide health benefits. Lipids will improve and insulin resistance will decrease.

No one should be seduced by these early changes. If you encourage your patient to eat a diet of flesh foods, the real issues become: What are you brewing up in their colon wall? In his prostate? In her breast tissue? What's happening in your patient's arteries? What's happening in their brain? *Do no harm* applies to dietary advice as well.

Healthcare tends to be very episodic: Patients who periodically drop into clinics seldom see the same doctor in the clinic upon return. Patients move away; doctors move away. Imagine some young doctor who casually recommends the Paleo diet. That doctor may never see the patient again.

But the patient follows that advice, and day after day, year after year, packs their intestines with meat and runs these toxins through their bloodstream. I would say to that young doctor who dispensed that drive-by dietary advice: "Are you going to be around in ten years when this man passes his bloody stool from the colon cancer your dietary advice cooked up in his colon? Are you going to be around in fifteen years when this woman has her stroke from the carotid plaque that your highly inflammatory diet produced in her carotid artery? Are you going to be around in twenty years when the Alzheimer's first starts setting in from the vascular changes your dietary advice promoted in this patient's brain? It's likely, Doc, that you won't be around to see it."

Therein lies the danger of this kind of casually dispensed, uninformed dietary advice. The arrogance involved in dispensing dietary advice without a solid understanding of nutrition should not be underestimated.

Food Changes Us

Food changes us in one of two ways. Either it changes us directly, epigenetically (turning our genes on and off), the way Neu5GC turns on inflammation, or it changes the microbes in our gut. And those microbes will change us, because they are not passive bystanders. Their byproducts include serotonin, oxytocin, norepinephrine, and dopamine; they put out these and other neurotransmitters that enter our brain and affect our mood and our perception. But either way, the food we eat changes us. It's often far more powerful in its effects than the drugs we prescribe. And yet, in virtually every aspect of medical education, we blow right past this powerful health-shaping force.

To practice medicine without regard to what your patient is eating puts a physician in the position of the blind men and the elephant. You may know the ancient parable: A group of blind men come upon an elephant and each takes hold of a different part of the great beast. One blind man grabs the trunk and thinks he has hold of a massive snake; one grabs the ear and believes the elephant is a broad fan; another, with his hand on the tail, thinks he has found a rope; one touches the side of the elephant and deems it a wall; and the tusk grabber assumes the elephant is a spear. They all have hold of the same elephant, but none has a clue what the whole elephant really is.

That's the predicament of the physician who practices without nutritional awareness. It is especially the case for our own beloved specialists, trying to decipher and treat the particular diseases they grapple with in their isolated bailiwicks. The cardiologist sees the clogged arteries; the internist sees the high blood pressure; the rheumatologist sees the lupus; the endocrinologist sees the type 2 diabetes; the gastroenterologist sees the Crohn's and the colitis; the dermatologist sees the psoriasis; the neurologist sees the stroke; the physiatrist sees the sore joints; the general surgeon sees the diverticulitis. They're all trying to figure out their own separate diseases. Yet, if they think about it, they would realize that all these diseases have some commonalities—they all have elements of inflammation, excessive production of free radicals, and high oxidative stress. It behooves them to ask: What factor could be inciting inflammation, excessive free-radical activity, and oxidative stress in all of these patients? Is there a common factor that each of them is exposed to?

I'd like to sneak quietly into their cubicles and yell smartly into their ears: *It's the food that your patients are eating! That's what is supplying these disruptive substances!*

Does our medical establishment, which refuses to question the animal food–based Western diet, or investigate its effects on our bodies, or counsel against its continued adoption, imagine that we are some outlier carnivorous primate? Surely those who run medical schools and hospitals know that we evolved on this planet up through the simian line. Primates have been on this planet for at least fifty million years, and they are—*we are*—by nature plant-eating creatures. We have fingers on our hands, not claws; we have long intestines for digesting fiber, not the short intestines of carnivores, efficient for ridding the body of decaying flesh. We humans have saliva with starch-digesting amylase, not protein-digesting proteases. We have the jaw structure and dentition of herbivores, not of carnivores or omnivores. Yes, our ancestors could scavenge a little flesh from time to time for survival purposes, but we were never meant to eat a flesh-based diet. We don't have a digestive system that remotely resembles that of mountain lions.

If you check out the Blue Zones, areas of the world where the highest percentages of centenarians live, you find that all of them are eating largely plant-based diets. None of those populations happen to be completely vegan; there's commonly a little bit of fish or other flesh foods in their diets. But the vast majority of what goes down their gullets grows out of the ground, and we should take a lesson from that.

Most of the medical profession does not. We continue to practice medicine as if what our patients eat has no effect on their health. It's an appalling, grotesque deficiency in medical education. It overlooks a basic fact of physiology: Within minutes of eating anything, molecules of that food flow through every cell in your body, where your DNA strands lie unfolded. As the food molecules wash across your DNA, they play your genes like a piano. They turn genes on; they turn genes off. They induce enzymes; they shut enzymes down. The content of each meal not only brings nutrients into our body, but it also brings in information. Every meal changes you on a genetic, molecular level. We cannot overlook that fact; the consequences to our health are too clear. You don't need to be a geneticist to understand that the genes that are going to be turned on by a grilled steak, with all the disrupting, contaminating molecules that it contains washing across your DNA and setting off everything from aging to autoimmunity to cancer, will be thoroughly different than the genes that will be turned on by a salad, which sends a surge of stabilizing phytonutrients—such as polyphenols and sulforaphanes—through your tissues. These phytonutrients are rich with antioxidants that quench free radicals, promote tissue repair, and send a calming chemical message to your tissues.

We can't pretend that a flesh-based meal doesn't have markedly different consequences to your body on a genetic and molecular level than a whole plant food meal. You may have a genetic propensity to develop diabetes or colon cancer, but whether that disease actually manifests in your body greatly depends on the molecules you're flushing through your tissues on a daily basis.

Every meal changes us. Food can create health, or it can contribute to disease. Doctors need to understand this and to act upon it. As a mechanism to reverse metabolic disorders, dietary therapy trumps all other approaches; indeed, the pharmaceutical approach often does not even attempt to reverse disease but only to control its effects. Physicians who overlook dietary therapy tie both hands behind their backs, and then they often struggle with the sense of helplessness that afflicted me in Vancouver. To address the metabolic disorders of the general population without the tool of dietary therapy makes no more sense than addressing acute appendicitis without the tool of surgery. Sure, it is possible, here and there, to treat appendicitis with antibiotics alone, especially for patients who are not good candidates for surgery. But no sane physician facing a patient in severe abdominal pain from acute appendicitis would or should adopt the *a priori* stance of a blanket opposition to surgical removal of the appendix, which is certainly the optimal solution for many, if not most, sufferers of appendicitis. Similarly, the optimal solution for most metabolic disorders is dietary change—often profound dietary change. And yet most physicians in our nation today dismiss this option out of hand.

Let me note here an important fact that makes this analogy particularly apt: A high-fiber diet rich in fruits and vegetables will—unsurprisingly to anyone with a basic understanding of nutrition, anatomy, and pathology (this should be a description of all doctors)—dramatically reduce your chances of developing appendicitis in the first place.[13]

Meal after meal, month after month, year after year, the Red Tide of toxins repeatedly surges through all the cells, eventually leading to such maladies as obesity, atherosclerosis, type 2 diabetes, hypertension, and many types of cancer.

This is a fundamental, undeniable fact that places metabolism squarely at the center of the universe of concerns affecting human health. This is something that practicing doctors and medical students must understand in order to become true healers.

We have to end the madness that is the medical ignorance of nutrition.

Chapter Three

UNDERSTANDING NUTRITIONAL THERAPY, PART ONE

Prevention and Reversal of Cardiovascular Disease, Type 2 Diabetes, and Hypertension

Let's consider the nature of disease. You can think of the word as dis-ease; the body is not at ease with itself. *Merriam-Webster* defines it as "a condition of the living animal or plant body or of one of its parts that impairs normal functioning and is typically manifested by distinguishing signs and symptoms."

When we hear that someone we know has developed a disease, we generally think of it as bad luck. Some unfortunate gene kicked in, and our poor friend now suffers from a condition that we thank our lucky stars we have not developed ourselves.

On the other hand, of course, if a friend who smokes two packs a day develops lung cancer, we are not surprised. In that case, we know very well that our friend has most likely smoked their way into their condition. And if we are not smokers, we don't need to waste time thanking our lucky stars. We didn't do anything "wrong" to bring on lung cancer.

The truth is that there are few diseases that lack a causal agent that we can identify. There are viral conditions like pneumonia, chicken pox, shingles, herpes, and polio, for which we can identify the viruses that bring them on. There are conditions like asthma, mesothelioma, and lead poisoning, for which we can often identify environmental causes.

And then there are the diseases that we discuss as if they are simply bad luck: heart disease, prostate cancer, breast cancer, high blood pressure, type 2 diabetes, and autoimmune conditions, to name a few.

The human body is not capricious. It doesn't wake up one day and decide: "It's a good time to brew up angina, or maybe high blood pressure." As a general rule, the body manifests these diseases only when our behavior enforces that outcome upon it.

To the slight extent that doctors in America evaluate their patients' diets at all, most do not allow themselves to follow the science. Instead, they follow the dictates of the culture, or at least they allow the culture to color their interpretation of the science. They do not even entertain the notion that animal foods should be eliminated from the human diet as pro-inflammatory substances. They do not concern themselves with the impact of animal foods on the human biome or the human bloodstream. They allow themselves to be fooled by the claims of the meat industry that animal protein offers some health advantage, when in fact the opposite is true: Animal protein will stress your kidneys and may even prove carcinogenic. Most doctors eat animal foods themselves, and therefore they do not even consider counseling their patients against doing the same. And so animal foods continue to wreak havoc upon our bodies.

Let us look now at some of the impacts they have on different health conditions, and how effectively their elimination from the human diet can contribute to health.

Prevention and Reversal of Cardiovascular Disease

In our overmedicalized society, it may seem that most adults you know take statin drugs to lower the cholesterol level in their blood. You might deduce that the human population has been suddenly cursed with genes that instruct our livers to crank out so much artery-clogging "bad" cholesterol that we have no recourse but to attach chemical brakes, in the form of statins, onto the enzymes in those errant livers that synthesize too much cholesterol.

This model holds that we are largely passive victims in the genetic lottery that doles out our cardiovascular risk according to our family history. The thinking goes that if your father died of heart disease, it's likely that you will, too. Evil ol' cholesterol seems to have become Public Enemy Number One of cardiologists and TV commercials alike; lowering your "bad" LDL number has turned into something of a national sport.

The Truth About Cholesterol

Why, you may ask, did Mother Nature saddle us with this lethal molecule that daily flows through our bloodstream, injuring our arteries, and eventually causing our early demise in a thunderclap of chest pain and sudden cardiac arrest? What was Her motivation? Was She not concerned with our capacity to survive in good health? Was She perhaps trying to kill us off before we could pave Her beautiful planet?

I would modestly submit that we might consider giving Mother Nature some credit. Let's recognize that cholesterol is not an evil molecule at all. As you read these words, your liver is delivering to your bloodstream cholesterol that has far more benevolent functions than generating atherosclerotic plaque in your artery walls; in fact, as a molecule produced within the context of a salubrious diet, cholesterol should not contribute to generating plaque at all.

Cholesterol is NOT an Evil Molecule

Your liver makes cholesterol for:
Adrenal steroid synthesis
Bile synthesis for fat absorbtion
Estrogen and testosterone synthesis
Cell membrane construction

The cholesterol molecule is a rather elegant structure, with three adjoining hexagonal rings, each composed of six atoms of carbon. One of the rings is connected to a fourth, pentagonal ring of five carbon atoms. From that five-carbon ring, there dangles a side chain of carbon atoms that can be shortened or altered by various organs to give the cholesterol molecule special properties, such as building muscle or helping to maintain a pregnancy.

Your adrenal glands—fatty organs shaped like a three-cornered hat, perched on top of your kidneys—take that cholesterol molecule, enzymatically shorten and reconfigure the side chain, and thereby create essential adrenocortical hormones, such as cortisol and its vital cousins, aldosterone and dehydroepiandrosterone (DHEA).

If you are a woman, your ovaries take that same cholesterol molecule, do some chemistry on the side groups, and turn cholesterol into the potent feminizing molecules, estrone and estradiol. If you are a man, your testicles transform cholesterol into testosterone. And every cell in your mammalian body uses cholesterol molecules to repair injuries to vital, but fragile, cell membranes.

Much of the public's confusion over cholesterol's role in the human body stems from a conflation of the required, natural cholesterol, which our own liver produces for vital bodily functions, with the foreign, unnatural *oxidized dietary cholesterol*, which comes from ingested animal foods. Remember that the animal foods to which we attach various names like "steak," "drumsticks," and "pork chops" are really the muscle tissues of cows, chickens, and pigs. All animal muscle contains cholesterol in abundance. The searing heat typically found in ovens, grills, and deep fryers easily tears electrons off cholesterol molecules, oxidizing them.

Cholesterol, therefore, in its native form as produced by the liver, is not a villain. But it is an easy molecule to oxidize. Small particles of low-density cholesterol (LDL-C) that have become oxidized are called *oxysterols*, such as 7-ketocholesterol, 7β-hydroxycholesterol, and 5,6-epoxycholesterol. These particles, each missing an electron, are, indeed, the seeds of the lethal plaque that eventually forms in the artery walls in most everyone who eats the standard Western diet, generating the disease of atherosclerosis.

While the cooking of meat at high temperatures plays a role in fostering plaque formation, there is an even more significant source of cholesterol oxidation. Most of the plaque-building, oxidized cholesterol in the artery walls is generated from small LDL cholesterol molecules in the blood that become sequestered in the artery walls, thanks to a special protein they carry on the particles' surface, called *Apolipoprotein B*, or *ApoB*. In fact, ApoB can be viewed as the most atherogenic particle, and the number of ApoB particles is currently seen as the best predictor of atherosclerotic plaque formation, more so than just the amount of LDL.

An animal-food-based diet will raise your ApoB number, as both saturated fat and dietary cholesterol increase the liver's production of ApoB-containing cholesterol, while the fiber attendant to a diet of whole plant foods helps to remove ApoB-containing cholesterol particles from the bloodstream via the stool.

We have seen that the LDL particles, sequestered in the matrix of the artery walls by their ApoB protein, are eventually oxidized into oxysterols by cellular enzymes in the subendothelial layers of the artery wall. There, the newly oxidized lipids ignite an inflammatory reaction that summons immune cells called *macrophages*, which promptly engulf the oxidized LDL particles. In feasting on the reactive oxysterol particles, the macrophages themselves become cauldrons of seething free-radical activity, secreting inflammatory cytokines into the surrounding tissues and further fanning the flames of inflammation in the artery walls. As they gorge upon the oxysterols, the macrophages take on a frothy appearance, hence the name "foam" cells.

The foam cells then accumulate and aggregate in the walls of the arteries, soon generating a significant atherosclerotic plaque. Each plaque contains a core made of oxidized cholesterol and cellular debris. It soon becomes infiltrated with lymphocytes and dendritic cells (specialized immune cells), and finally it's sealed with a cap made of smooth muscle cells and fibroblasts (cells that help create connective tissue).

Under repeated onslaughts of Red Tide toxins, including oxysterols generated by the cooking of meat that fans the inflammatory process, the plaques grow ever larger and can eventually encroach into the blood-flow channel. A large plaque can choke down blood flow through a key artery just when muscle fibers need that blood flow most, such as when the owner of the arteries is, say, running for a bus. At that moment, the maximally working muscles in the heart and leg muscles can find themselves shortchanged of vital, oxygen-carrying blood, which results in the crushing chest pain of angina pectoris and/or the deep, viselike ache in the leg's now-hypoxic muscles, called *claudication*.

The worst consequence transpires when a plaque softens and ruptures, exposing the ragged core of cholesterol to the bloodstream. The cells that initiate blood clotting—the platelets—contact the cholesterol core and are torn open. When they then release their enzymes and proteins, a clot can form on the surface of the plaque. Within minutes, that clot can grow to a size that obstructs the entire blood-flow channel, choking off vital oxygen and nutrients to the cells downstream. Those cells promptly die. If they are muscle cells in the heart, a heart attack—often causing a lethal arrhythmia—results; if the clot cuts off blood flow to nerve cells in the brain, those cells die, and a stroke is the usual outcome.

It is often, but not always, the case that, before the dreadful happens in the form of a heart attack or a stroke, the owner of the afflicted arteries experiences symptoms. When the muscle cells are starved of blood flow, oxygen levels drop, and lactic acid accumulates in the heart muscle tissues, bringing on the crushing chest pain of angina pectoris, which soon becomes unbearable.

You do not want to experience the awful sensation of angina; it is not only painful but also laden with the premonition of one's own death. Angina's message is: "This is likely how you will die." In angina's grip, your death now has a shape, a feel, a presence. It is an awful sensation to live with.

The end, in the form of a vascular death, often does, indeed, come eventually. The muscle fibers of the heart, starved of oxygen and nutrients, begin to die (infarct). If many heart muscle fibers are suddenly infarcted, the area in the wall of the heart surrounding the infarction becomes electrically unstable. The injured cells send out random electrical impulses, disrupting normal heart rhythms and producing dire effects upon the amount of blood being pumped. Instead of pumping in a coordinated, controlled manner, the fibers begin to quiver randomly (the phenomenon known as *fibrillation*). If this happens in the wall of one of the main pumping chambers (the left or right ventricle), forward propulsion of blood to the brain, kidneys, and heart muscle itself ceases, potentially bringing a sudden end to life—the mode of exit from this world for about one thousand Americans, and about 150 Canadians, every day.[1]

Healing a Damaged Artery

Is artery clogging from atherosclerotic plaque a relentlessly progressive process, inevitably leading to a cardiac catastrophe? Most cardiologists think so, and that is understandable. After all, that's what they were taught in medical school. Furthermore, unless the doctor can prevail upon their patient to modify their food stream into one that stops the ongoing damage, this is exactly what the physician and the patient will witness.

But it doesn't have to be that way, as Dr. Caldwell B. Esselstyn Jr., a surgeon at the Cleveland Clinic, has conclusively demonstrated.

Dr. Esselstyn provided dramatic evidence in 2014 of how reversible this process can be. In a landmark pilot study,[2] he describes 198 patients (180 men; 18 women), each of whom had severe atherosclerosis. Each person had suffered either a myocardial infarction, a stroke, and/or episodes of angina pectoris. The entire arterial trees of these people were so clogged up with plaque, there was no workable place to insert a stent. Coronary artery bypass grafts could not be accomplished because there were no "normal" arterial segments into which a venous bypass graft could be connected. These patients were regarded as having "end-stage" vascular disease and thus fell beyond the limits of standard therapy. Therefore, when Dr. Esselstyn announced his study on just such patients, his cardiologist colleagues were more than happy to ship off those who were not candidates for aggressive intervention—namely, surgery or stenting—to his "conservative" protocol. I say "conservative" because his protocol involved no risky procedures or untested drugs; it did involve, however, a "radical" change in diet.

Dr. Esselstyn's protocol had these patients consume a diet of whole plant foods, with very little fat: no meat, dairy, or other animal products, as well as no oils, avocado, or nuts, because of the adverse effects of these fatty plant foods upon the endothelial lining of the blood vessels that were so in need of healing. Refined grains and excess sugars were also discouraged. This dietary maneuver was extremely potent, with its most important effect being the cessation of the repeated Red Tides. A diet of nothing but whole plant foods delivers respite, at last, from the recurring floods of molecular marauders—such as oxidized cholesterol, uric acid, advanced glycation end products, and free radicals—carried to tissues in a fatty, meat-marred bloodstream. There was now opportunity for healing on a cellular level to begin, with a more free-flowing, healthier bloodstream efficiently delivering antioxidants and phytonutrients that enhance cellular repair.

Every cell, every tissue, and, thus, every organ in our body has built-in repair mechanisms to keep the cellular machinery functioning smoothly. We all have DNA-editing enzymes inside our DNA strands looking for damage and mismatched nucleotides. And when they find such errors, they correct them. What a remarkable system! When I first read about this in a medical text, I put my book down and applauded. To think we have such potent molecular allies in every cell, looking after us, keeping us healthy, and functioning optimally, truly is cause for awe and wonder.

Still, these amazing mini healers cannot efficiently perform their repair work if, every four hours, another surge of Red Tide toxins sweeps through the cells and inhibits their cellular repair. However, when fortified and protected by a phytonutrient-rich, whole plant food diet, like that utilized by Dr. Esselstyn's program, the repair proteins can go about their restorative tasks uninhibited and begin to return the function of the artery walls to normal. Artery walls with healthy, intact endothelial linings can generate sufficient amounts of nitric oxide (NO) to keep the muscular walls flexible. This is an important trait, allowing the arteries to absorb much of the jolt of energy that gets transmitted down the blood-flow column with every heartbeat. If this pulsatile energy is not absorbed and "softened" by elastic artery walls, this pulse wave can damage delicate tissues downstream, such as the capillaries in the retinas of the eyes, which could lead to retinal hemorrhages and, at worst, blindness.

Among the most dramatic findings in Dr. Esselstyn's study was this: The lethal plaques themselves began to melt away. How could this be? The formation of plaques was deemed (and still is, by most cardiologists) to be a one-way, irreversible process. Yet, evidence that such a remarkable reversal of atherosclerotic plaque accumulation was indeed happening became evident in the study of these 198 patients over four years. Had they followed the usual clinical course of American men with vascular disease who continue to eat the Standard American Diet, statistically, sixty of these men would have been expected to suffer a major adverse cardiac event (MACE) in the form of a myocardial infarction, a stroke, a cardiac arrest episode, or sudden death over the span of four years. As it turned out, 177 of the 198 patients remained compliant with the diet. How many of these compliant patients suffered a MACE in four years? Answer: one (he suffered a stroke). Yet, in the group of patients who were *not* compliant with Dr. Esselstyn's diet (there were twenty-one such subjects, of the 198 in the study), 62 percent (thirteen of them) suffered a MACE during the same four years.[3]

As further indication of artery healing, including plaque resolution, 93 percent of the diet-compliant subjects who had suffered from angina had their chest pain upon exertion markedly improve or resolve altogether on Dr. Esselstyn's program.

Why did Dr. Esselstyn's program achieve such spectacular results? The possible mechanisms explaining the dramatic disease reversal of arterial plaque on Dr. Esselstyn's plant-only program are many:

- the lack of repeated Red Tide assaults, filled with AGEs and oxidized cholesterol
- the return of endogenous repair mechanisms
- the abundant antioxidants that quench free radicals in the artery walls
- the lack of gut microbes that generate atherogenic TMAO (trimethylamine N-oxide)
- the increased production of nitric oxide in arterial endothelium that restores arterial elasticity and function

These benevolent forces, at work 24/7, week after week, in Dr. Esselstyn's patients, eventually turned the tide on this otherwise lethal disease.

One of the secrets to the success of the program may be found in Dr. Esselstyn's insistence that every participant consume a fist-size helping of dark-green vegetables, such as kale, collard greens, bok choy, brussels sprouts, and broccoli, at least four or five times per day! He also recommended that they "anoint" the greens with a tablespoon of balsamic vinegar before consuming them.

What was behind this strategy? The constant, or nearly constant, presence of a bolus of dark-green vegetables in the small intestine permits that digested food to function as a time-release capsule of antioxidant molecules, effectively keeping a steady level of these free radical–neutralizing substances in the bloodstream, twenty-four hours a day. Over time, the ever-present antioxidant molecules in the blood flow seep their way into the walls of the arteries and into the atherosclerotic plaques. There, they neutralize the swarm of free radicals in the plaques, quenching any oxidative fires in the artery walls.

With no free radicals keeping the plaques inflamed, swollen, and unstable, the focal adhesions holding the plaque together are broken, so foam cells regain their mobility and out-migrate from the plaque. *Voila!*—plaques begin to resorb, or break apart, and more open arteries result.

How about that damaged endothelium on the artery walls? Could that be repaired? Strikingly, the answer again is yes. Here is where that balsamic vinegar works its salubrious effects: The polyphenols in the vinegar stimulate nitric oxide synthase enzymes in the endothelium that produce nitric oxide, thus promoting repair of that essential membrane.

As the plaque melts away from the inner surface of the arteries, and the muscular walls of the arterial tubing regain their elasticity from the restored nitric oxide function, a subtle vasodilation can now occur. This enlarges the blood-flow channel by a small amount. However, that small increase in the bore of the artery makes a big difference when it comes to oxygen delivery to the tissues, thanks to a law in physics known as *Poiseuille's law.*

Poiseuille's Law

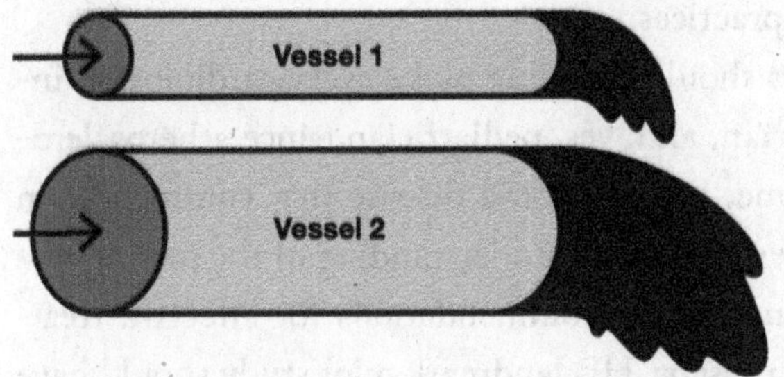

$$Q = \frac{\Delta P \pi r^4}{8 \eta l}$$

A small increase in the width of the pipe means a very large increase in flow through the pipe.

Increase the radius by a factor of two, and the flow increases by a factor of sixteen.

This principle states that the flow of liquid through a pipe (think blood flowing through an artery) will increase by the fourth power of the increase of the radius. That means that the melting away of even some of the restricting plaque, combined with a small degree of vasodilation from the increased nitric oxide production in the endothelium, will greatly increase the flow of blood in the artery. By how much? If the radius of the cross section of the artery increased by merely 10 percent, the flow of blood would increase to the fourth power of 1.1, which is 1.464—in other words, by more than 46 percent! So, a modest increase in the diameter of the artery delivers a highly significant increase in blood flow.

The extra water—now in the bloodstream from all the high-water-content food in the WPF diet (for example, cooked grains, soups, stews, salads, fruits, and smoothies)—facilitates vital blood flow even more. It has been demonstrated that vegetarians have blood that is measurably less viscous, so their blood is more free-flowing through vital capillary beds.[4]

Since atherosclerosis restricts arterial flow throughout the body, the plaque regression and resulting increased blood perfusion bring welcome relief to every organ. There is often return or improvement in kidney function, walking distance, visual acuity, and erectile function.

Or, as most men would read that last sentence: "There is often return or improvement in erectile function."

If Westerners did not eat a diet rich in animal products, oil, and sugar, then atherosclerosis—our society's biggest killer—would all but disappear. Plaque need never form in the walls of healthy arteries. When an unhealthy diet brings it on, however, it is clearly reversible with the appropriate dietary and lifestyle practices.

Dr. Esselstyn's findings should therefore make every cardiologist, internist, primary care physician, and, yes, pediatrician (since atherosclerosis has unfortunately become, in America, a disease that commences in childhood) immediately reevaluate their understanding of the pathophysiology of atherosclerosis and their recommendations for effective treatment to reverse any plaque present. His landmark pilot study should have prompted large-scale field research funded by the National Heart, Lung, and Blood Institute, part of the National Institutes of Health (NIH), to duplicate and perhaps even expand upon his findings. Instead, the reaction of the medical establishment to Dr. Esselstyn's staggering, groundbreaking study was silence. That made my heart sink. After all, Dr. Esselstyn had effectively afforded the NIH the opportunity to investigate and consequently promote a clear and obvious path to making heart disease—our most prolific killer—all but vanish, while at the same time dramatically improving the health of virtually all Americans in countless other ways.

But perhaps it is too much to hope that the NIH would view that outcome as relevant to its mission.

What Does All This Mean for You?

We can now reframe the classic questions about atherosclerosis. We now see that the question is not "How high is your cholesterol level?" but rather "How healthy are your artery walls?" In other words: "Do you have plaque forming in your arteries or don't you?" Those are the questions that anyone who has been eating the Standard American Diet needs to have answered.

Since we now know that the formation of atherosclerotic plaques in the artery walls always involves a degree of inflammation, testing the blood for markers of inflammation may be, for those who are concerned, worth doing. The most practical markers to test for—as is now commonly done by many commercial testing laboratories—are:

1. LDL cholesterol, with ApoB estimation
2. High-sensitivity C-reactive protein (HS-CRP)
3. Myeloperoxidase (an enzyme that white blood cells use to soften plaque; this is a sign of plaque instability)
4. Lp(a)—a genetically determined form of cholesterol that promotes plaque formation and blood clotting. A WPF diet can mitigate many of its adverse effects, but if Lp(a) is elevated over

50 mg/dL or 125 nmol/L, consult a cardiologist for possible treatment strategies. Unfortunately, in rare cases, diet alone cannot protect you from a severely elevated Lp(a) score, and medication may be necessary.

To complete the picture, the carotid arteries in the neck can be examined by a safe, painless ultrasound scan, a radiation-free imaging technique that will give visual evidence as to whether plaque is present in the artery wall or not.

If your inflammatory markers in your blood are positive, and the ultrasound scan shows ragged plaque or thickening of the inner linings of the arteries, then you have the disease of atherosclerosis smoldering in your blood vessels, and the wisest course of action would be to jump onto Dr. Esselstyn's plaque-reversal program posthaste! You should also consult a cardiologist to see if a course of statins or another cholesterol-reducing agent may be warranted.

If the inflammatory markers in your blood are *not* positive, and the ultrasound scan shows no plaque and clean arteries, even if your blood cholesterol levels are moderately elevated, then the inflammatory fire of atherosclerosis is not burning in your arterial walls at this time. It is evidently possible for potentially atherogenic particles to flow through the bloodstream without causing artery damage, to be eventually removed, dismantled, and excreted by the liver.

If you are not yet eating a WPF diet but receive the welcome news that the inflammatory markers in your blood are not positive, and your ultrasound scan shows no plaque and clean arteries, you should consider yourself lucky. But realize that your luck may not hold. The wisest course of action would again be to adopt a diet of whole plant foods posthaste!

Therefore, since the optimal response will be the same regardless of the test results, it would not be illogical, *if you are not suffering any concerning symptoms*, and especially if you also want to save money and time, to simply forgo a raft of tests and adopt, with conviction, consistency, and determination, a diet of whole plant foods. If, however, you are already suffering concerning symptoms, it may be wiser to get yourself tested in case more needs to be done in the short term to protect your health than dietary change alone.

There may be occasions where a course of statin therapy is warranted until the artery inflammation subsides, but that should be determined by each patient and their cardiologist or family doctor. That said, even if statins are instituted, it should be done with an understanding that the medications may only be needed for six to eighteen months, after which retesting should be done. If clear signs of plaque reversal and inflammation subsidence are observed, and the Esselstyn-style, WPF diet is rigorously maintained, the statins can often be safely discontinued, with the patient regularly followed with blood tests and ultrasound scans until both doctor and patient are assured that the atherosclerotic fires have been extinguished in the artery walls. Unlike the way in which it is currently generally used, statin therapy need not be a lifetime prescription.

Where, you may ask, does the "calcium score" fit into all of this? This is a test often recommended by cardiologists. What is calcium doing in the artery walls, anyway? If an inflammatory process anywhere in the body continues for many months—say, a tendon sheath rubbing against a bone spur, or a bursa on the front of a knee continually knelt upon—the body's "Plan B" is to pack the affected tissues full of calcium, extinguishing the inflammatory fire by turning the tissues to stone. This is also true of the inflammatory process of atherosclerotic plaque formation in the walls of the arteries.

After years of inflammation smoldering unabated in and around the plaques slowly growing in the subendothelial layers of the artery walls, the body can call in the "cellular plasterers" to petrify the process and extinguish the inflammation. Flecks of calcium begin to be deposited in the inflammatory cells surrounding and within the atherosclerotic plaque. Over time, the calcifications grow and coalesce with each other, forming a calcium cast of the artery wall. There is an important trade-off involved in this process: On the positive side, calcified plaques are no longer in danger of rupturing and unleashing a clot. On the other hand, the artery becomes less pliable and the blood-flow channel is often permanently narrowed.

The calcium flecks are easily seen on a CT scan of the chest, allowing a "calcium score" to be determined. Larger amounts of calcium deposited—a high calcium score—correlates with a more severe atherosclerotic inflammation that has been present in the artery wall. This score is taken as a predictive risk factor in having a MACE. People who have a high calcium score stand at risk of a MACE if they continue eating the standard fatty Western diet and continue injuring their arteries three times a day with the Red Tide toxic trespassers. But what is the calcium score really telling us?

Long ago, I visited Gettysburg National Military Park and found, in the visitor center, a huge diorama bedecked with hundreds of small plaster soldiers, half of them painted in Union blue and half in Confederate gray. Each soldier stood in a pose of battle with his rifle, bayonet, or pistol. These inert plaster soldiers, frozen in time, signified the furious battle in the past. In the same way, we can view the calcium flecks in the artery walls as remnants of the inflammatory fire that burned in the walls of the arteries some time ago.

The calcified plaques themselves do not pose any significant threat to their owner, as they are petrified, and thus stable. They won't rupture, and so they will not set off a clot and cause a myocardial infarction. A person's calcium score will never decrease, however, even if their health improves according to many other metrics. The calcium buttressing is simply not going anywhere, and we don't want it to. It is performing an important function in preventing rupture of the plaque.

The message of the calcification, however, is not to be ignored. A significant calcium score announces loud and clear that there has been a roaring fire of inflammation in the walls of the arteries. If nothing has changed in the person's diet, that roaring fire is undoubtedly going to continue blazing. The owner of those arteries should therefore seriously consider immediately adopting an anti-inflammatory diet and lifestyle before a soft plaque—the kind that does not show up on a CT scan and is likely present—*does* rupture and set off that lethal clot we all fear. By adopting a whole plant food diet from that point on, every meal promotes healing instead of advancing disease.

What is lost in the calcium score is that people who have a high calcium score stand at risk of a MACE *if they continue eating the Standard American Diet and continue injuring their arteries three times a day with the Red Tide dietary disruptors.*

The issue isn't only with the artery wall but also with the smoothness of the blood-flow channel on the inside of the arteries, including the health and velvety integrity of the endothelial membrane.

Fortunately, the endothelial membrane constantly heals and renews itself, thanks to a steady shower of stem cells from the bone marrow that land on the endothelium and begin to patch any abraded areas and restore smooth blood flow. People with high calcium scores who adopt an Esselstyn-style WPF diet can heal the inner blood-flow channel and write a different cardiac future for themselves.

So, if you have not already had a CT scan looking for calcium deposited in the walls of your coronary arteries, and you have already committed to consuming a whole plant food diet, do you need to obtain such a scan? There is a classic adage that every young physician learns to consider when ordering medical tests on any patient: "If it's not going to change your treatment, don't order the test." By far, the most effective therapy for lowering cholesterol and arresting the progression of atherosclerotic vascular disease is adoption of, and adherence to, a WPF diet. One should adopt this strategy immediately, regardless of cholesterol numbers, calcium score, or even symptoms such as angina (yes, angina pectoris is reversible). It is never unsafe nor too early to begin melting away plaques in the artery walls with a low- or moderate-fat WPF diet.

That said, if your LDL cholesterol is well over 130 mg/dL (3.4–4.1 mmol/L), if your ApoB level exceeds 80 mg/dL (800 nmol/L), or if your Lp(a) exceeds 50 mg/dL (125 nmol/L)—and, especially, if you are experiencing any cardiac symptoms, such as irregular heartbeat or angina pectoris upon exertion—you will want to consult a cardiologist to discuss medications to lower the risks these unique molecules present. Yet, despite the presence of these problematic substances, an artery-soothing WPF diet still makes sense for its higher water content, lack of pro-inflammatory foods such as refined carbohydrates and saturated fats, lack of dietary cholesterol, and abundant supplies of antioxidants and endothelium-healing nitric oxide precursors. The WPF diet and the resulting weight loss that usually accompanies it can lower ApoB levels,[5] thus significantly augmenting the benefits of any medications that may be prescribed.

You should understand that most cardiologists, suffering woefully from a lack of nutritional understanding, believe their patients will need to continue taking statins for the rest of their lifetime. Therefore, those who adopt the Esselstyn plaque-reversal program should work with their physician to follow their inflammatory markers and ultrasound scans of their carotid arteries for signs of inflammation subsidence and plaque resolution. Once these processes are solidly underway, discussions should be had regarding tapering off the statins over six to eighteen months. You may need to educate your cardiologist about why your inflammatory markers, lipid panels, and ultrasound scan images are improving! Be aware that there is often a transient rebound elevation of total cholesterol for a few months after statin cessation, but it should be viewed as benign and not contributing to plaque deposition if the whole plant food diet is maintained.

(NOTE: A patient who experiences angina pain while at rest may be building up to a full-blown heart attack; that situation should be evaluated by a cardiologist immediately, and more significant interventions may be called for.)

Are longtime vegans immune to developing atherosclerotic plaques in their arteries? That depends on the type of vegan diet they practice. If they are practicing a WPF diet, free of added salt, oil, and sugar, and their total cholesterol is below 150 mg/dL (3.8 mmol/L), then the odds of their developing significant arterial plaque becomes vanishingly small.

In my practice, I have seen three twenty-year vegans develop significant angina. All three of them had been eating diets that, while vegan, clearly were not artery friendly. One had a sweet tooth and often ate vegan donuts, cupcakes, cookies, and other pastries. He also cooked with vegetable oils and ate fried foods liberally—practices decidedly not artery friendly. The fructose in the sweeteners used in these pastries and the toxic vegetable oils in the fried foods delivered a one-two punch to the vascular endothelium.

My second vegan angina patient was a bachelor who traveled frequently for his job and ate most every meal in restaurants. He did his best to order animal-free entrees, but, in reality, his food stream was a high-fat, high-sugar river of processed foods, soft drinks, vegan cheeses, and late-night chips. His arteries responded to this assault with atherosclerotic plaques in his coronary and carotid arteries.

My third vegan patient, thinking that fruit juice must be healthy, drank liters of apple juice daily for years, exposing his artery walls and liver cells to, no doubt, unhealthy levels of problematic sugars, especially fructose. In response to the toxic amounts of fructose, his liver became fatty and his artery walls developed plaque. He had become a vegan originally because of his love for animals. As sweet as it might be if this were the case, your arteries do not reward you merely for loving animals. They reward you for eating the diet of whole plant foods that humans evolved to eat. All three of these vegans are now on long-term statin treatments, and each has had coronary artery stents placed for their stubborn angina pectoris.

The experiences of these three vegans serve as cautionary tales for other vegans who contact me more often than you might suppose with concerns about their elevated cholesterol levels. They ask, "If I have been vegan for all these years, why is my cholesterol up and what should I do about it?" I first point out that, as we age, the liver becomes less efficient at removing LDL from the bloodstream, and so cholesterol levels naturally tend to rise with the years, but this likely does not pose a threat to the healthy WPF eater. I also counsel them, however, to take an honest look at what they've been eating. If they've been eating oils, either used in sautéing vegetables, added to salad dressings, or hidden in baked goods, eliminating those oils should be the first change they make. High consumption of vegan baked goods and sweets, ripe bananas, fruit juices, and dried fruits can also raise cholesterol levels in sugar-sensitive individuals, due to a surge of insulin to cope with high sugar levels.[6]

Fructose is unlike other sugars; the body does not metabolize it in the same way as it does glucose, which acts as a fuel for all our cells. Glucose in whole plant foods and fructose in its natural fruit forms will not turn into fat; but isolated fructose, when consumed in excess, is the one sugar that the body *can* turn into fat. Some fructose is metabolized in the liver as a source of energy for that vital organ; but beyond that, excess fructose will be transformed by the liver into triglycerides and uric acid. High triglycerides in turn contribute to high cholesterol levels. High uric acid levels can contribute to gout and can lead to kidney stones. The uric acid can also dock with receptors for advanced glycation end products (RAGEs) on the artery walls and produce inflammation that can promote plaque formation.

Impact of Excessive Fructose in the Diet

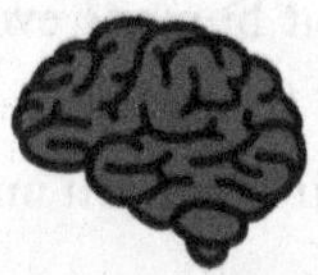
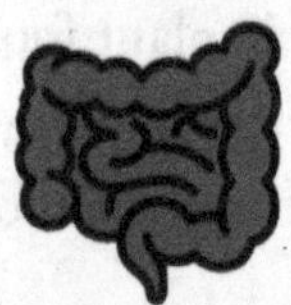
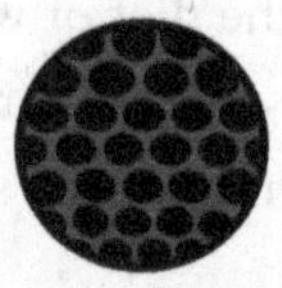
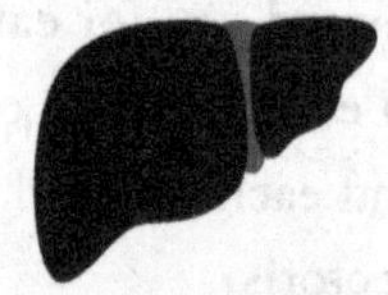

Central Nervous System	Intestine	Adipose Tissue	Liver
Causes leptin resistance Decreases satiety Decreases postprandial suppression of ghrelin Increases fructosylation of proteins Disrupts brain metabolism	Alters intestinal barrier integrity Alters microbial composition and functions	Induces obesity Induces inflammation Induces insulin resistance	Increases lipogenesis Decreases lipid oxidation Reduces ATP and uric acid formation Increases inflammation and cellular stress Decreases insulin sensitivity Activates hepatic stellate cell and upregulates fibrosis

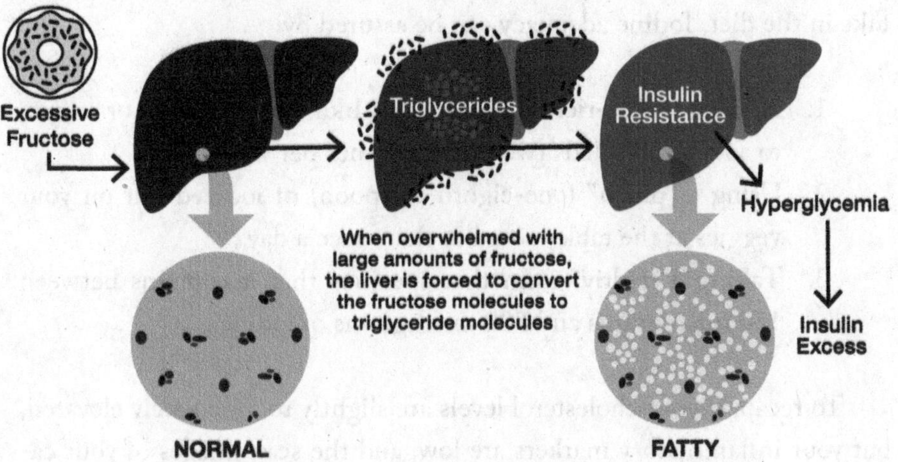

Excess fructose is converted by the liver into triglycerides, leading to insulin resistance.

Then we must consider the companion food to sugar in so many processed foods, including those eaten by vegans: oil. Even in olive oil, so often praised by fans of the Mediterranean diet, about 14 percent of the fat is saturated,[7] and, like most saturated fats, it can inhibit the liver's ability to remove cholesterol from the blood, thus contributing to hypercholesterolemia.

For most vegans with high cholesterol, ridding the diet of oils and excessive junk sugars in soft drinks, baked goods, and other sweetened, processed foods usually does the trick, permitting cholesterol levels to tumble to safer ranges within a few weeks' time.

If that doesn't work, the long-term vegan with consistently elevated cholesterol levels (over 250 mg/dL) may need to have a blood test for familial hypercholesterolemia (FH), a genetic disorder. Another common cause of stubbornly elevated cholesterol levels is low thyroid function (hypothyroidism), which may result from damage to the thyroid gland from sleep deprivation, a sedentary lifestyle, cigarette smoking, or alcohol abuse. We all would benefit by ridding ourselves of these artery saboteurs.

Another potential cause of low thyroid function is insufficient iodine intake in the diet. Iodine adequacy can be assured by:

1. Adding iodine-rich sea vegetables, like wakame, nori, or arame, to soups and salads two or three times per week
2. Using a "pinch" (one-eighth teaspoon) of iodized salt on your veggies at the table, no more than once a day
3. Taking a multivitamin that specifies that it contains between 150 micrograms and 500 micrograms of iodine

To recap, if your cholesterol levels are slightly to moderately elevated, but your inflammatory markers are low, and the scan images of your carotid arteries are pristine, then one can deduce that the inflammatory fires of plaque formation are not smoldering in your arteries. You should just carry on with your artery-friendly lifestyle: practicing a WPF diet; avoiding smoking, alcohol, and drug use; maintaining an optimal weight; getting reasonable daily exercise such as taking regular walks; spending some time in nature; and getting adequate sleep. You would want to recheck your inflammatory markers and artery scans every few years to learn if there is any plaque formation brewing—and take the appropriate steps we have discussed if it is found.

Dr. Esselstyn once wrote these words that I hope young cardiologists will take to heart:

> It is increasingly a shameful national embarrassment for the United States to have constructed a billion-dollar cardiac healthcare industry surrounding an illness that does not even exist in more than half of the planet. . . . We ignore CVD inception initiated by progressive endothelial injury, inflammatory oxidative stress, decreased nitric oxide production, foam cell formation, diminished endothelial progenitor cell production and development of plaque that may rupture and cause myocardial infarction or stroke. This series of events is primarily set in

> motion, and worsened, by the Western diet, which consists of added oils, dairy, meat, fish, fowl, and sugary foods and drinks—all of which injure endothelial function after ingestion, making food a major, if not the major cause of CAD.[8]

In light of Dr. Esselstyn's words, and knowing how preventable and even reversible this killer disease has proven to be in the face of a WPF diet accompanied by positive lifestyle practices, the question must be put to cardiologists and, indeed, to all physicians: Do you want to heal these people or to just manage their chronic disease? The doctors who choose the latter course will find their medical practices transformed into a kind of prolonged dirge, as they preside over the predictable demise of patients who dig their graves with their forks.

Prevention and Reversal of Type 2 Diabetes

If one could taste the spectrum of disease in American society, it would have a sickly-sweet flavor to it. This is because at any given hour, almost half the people you meet on Main Street in the United States are walking around with an elevated level of sugar in their blood.

The healthiest fasting blood glucose levels are deemed to be in the 70 mg/dL to 99 mg/dL range. (Dr. Casey Means, in her book *Good Energy*, posits that the optimal fasting blood glucose level is 70–85 mg/dL,[9] and I do not disagree, although I would not diagnose prediabetes until I saw a fasting insulin level over 12 microunits µU/mL, which is a sign of insulin resistance—and, thus, prediabetes—that can appear well before we see a rise in fasting blood sugar.)

One can also diagnose prediabetes by a *chronically* elevated blood sugar. An elevated HgbA1c, namely between 5.7% and 6.4%, puts the person in the "prediabetes" range, and the dire news is that, as of 2021, approximately 97.6 million US adults age eighteen years or older are walking around with prediabetes—that is, with blood sugars that average over 117 mg/dL.[10] We can calculate that because their HgbA1c value tells us that at least 5.7% of their hemoglobin is sticky with sugar. To saturate 5.7% of your hemoglobin with sugar, you must have been maintaining an average glucose level of 117 mg/dL in your blood. As if determined to show where prediabetes can lead, an additional 37.3 million Americans have actual diabetes, meaning that their HgbA1c is over 6.5%, so they are walking around with an average blood sugar of at least 140 mg/dL.[11] Add these two populations together and we have almost 135 million Americans whose sugary-sweet blood puts them at risk for a host of gruesome injuries to their eyes, kidneys, heart, liver, arteries, and virtually every other organ in their body.

Of course, the level of glucose in the bloodstream is not constant. It rises after eating any food containing carbohydrates. The glucose level then falls as insulin, secreted by the pancreas, moves glucose out of the bloodstream into the cells to be burned for energy. That is why the most significant test for those with prediabetes or diabetes is the HgbA1c test, which measures the percentage of your hemoglobin that is sticky with sugar, from which we can calculate your average blood sugar levels over a period of two to three months.

On the Standard American Diet, the cells of the muscles and liver have become resistant to insulin's message to let sugar molecules enter, so the elevated sugar levels in the blood linger for hours.

How, exactly, does keeping an elevated level of sugar in your blood, day after day, inflict damage? Well, in the same way that an old-fashioned sugar cube placed in a saucer in which coffee has been spilled will draw the coffee up into the sugar mass by the capillary pull of the concentrated sugar, elevated glucose in the bloodstream can pull water out of the delicate membranes in your eyes, kidneys, and artery linings. In doing so, it can severely damage the delicate tissues that these organs rely upon to function. For this reason, carrying 117 mg/dL or more of sugar in your bloodstream, hour after hour, puts one squarely in the category of prediabetes, which is known to raise the risk of:

1. Atherosclerotic plaque clogging the arteries, increasing the risk of heart attacks
2. Hypertension (high blood pressure), increasing the risk of stroke and heart failure
3. Chronic kidney disease, as delicate glomerular filter membranes are injured
4. Nerve damage (neuropathy) that can create unremitting, "hot" neuritic pain in the legs
5. Eye disorders, such as diabetic retinopathy, that can lead to blindness
6. Fatty liver disease, which can result in cirrhosis and liver failure
7. Infections in many organs, especially the bladder and skin, as high sugar levels impair immune system function
8. Impaired wound healing, as high sugar levels in the tissues inhibit collagen-producing enzymes and thereby retard new skin formation
9. Skin disorders, such as fungal infections and hyperpigmentation (acanthosis nigricans)
10. Sleep apnea from fat accumulation around the neck and dysregulation of autonomic nerve function that may produce sagging and collapse of upper airway muscles
11. Generation of advanced glycation end products (AGEs) that damage proteins throughout the body through free-radical damage
12. Development of full-blown diabetes as beta cells continue to die off from the free radicals that chronic hyperglycemia generates

Why is this metabolic disorder happening? When people think of the cause of diabetes, they reflexively blame sugar consumption. The intuitive response is to eat a diet low in carbohydrates, in order to reduce sugar levels. Yet we are sugar-burning organisms. In our cells, glucose reigns as the preferred fuel for the energy-producing mitochondria. It was the carbohydrates in the form of starchy roots, tubers, wild legumes, grasses, and berries that, as ancient foragers for calories, our ancestors sought out and ate. The glucose these foods provide gets stored as glycogen in our muscles and liver. Then, when physical activity demands muscular movement, the glycogen is transformed by glycogenolysis into free glucose, which is shoveled into our mitochondria to be burned for energy. The cycle is never-ending: Starches and sugars are eaten and stored as glycogen. Think of energy in a rechargeable battery: Physical activity draws down on the store of burnable carbohydrates as we seek out more supplies of energy. When we then eat the next trove of fruits and starches, the glycogen stores are replenished—and so it goes. Fats stored in the body are kept for when the recurring supply of glucose becomes interrupted for forty-eight hours or more. But fat is an emergency fuel, meant to tide us over until the carbohydrate river resumes.

The body hoards fats for a reason. Fats are energy rich, but naturally occurring fats are rare and could not be depended upon by our ancestors. Even game animals, when they could be caught, were lean creatures, providing fewer calories in fats than the fat-marbled cows and pigs of today. So unless your ancestors lived under an avocado or olive tree, fats were a relative rarity in their daily diet. Those advocates of the Paleo and keto approaches who argue that a high-fat diet was the "natural" diet of humans do not grasp the realities of what nature provides in the way of calories for mammals. Our Paleo ancestors did not live in a world where fats were abundant and easy to gorge on.

It is no accident that when we eat sweet foods, our taste buds reward us with a pleasure-reinforcing pulse of dopamine. We love sweetness. We crave it, and that can be a good thing when it propels us to eat fruits. Glucose is not inherently evil, but many people have problems metabolizing it, leading them into the sugary swamp of chronic elevated blood glucose levels and, eventually, to full-blown diabetes. Why do those blood glucose levels remain elevated for hours after the sugary or doughy treat is long forgotten?

Is it because, as a society, we have suddenly been cursed with a population-wide inability to metabolize sugars? Have our genes changed? Or is it the sheer amount of sugar that Americans consume: sixty pounds (twenty-seven kilograms) per year per American,[12] translating to some seventeen teaspoons of sugar every day in the soft drinks, energy drinks, fruit juices, cereals, baked goods, candies, candy bars, yogurt, ice cream, instant oatmeal, salad dressings, and condiments, as well as added to coffee and tea?

No, we haven't lost our innate ability to metabolize sugars, and yes, the obscene quantity of refined sugars in the American diet is certainly a serious part of the problem. Refined sugar (in the form of cane sugar, brown sugar, high-fructose corn syrup, agave syrup, maple syrup, coconut sugar, and other processed sugar sources), stripped of all fiber, adds about three hundred nutrition-free calories to the daily diet of the average American, while contributing to obesity, fatty liver disease, heart disease, and dental caries. Free sugars (sugars stripped of their fiber) have also been linked to cancers and even to depression and cognitive impairment.[13] They can even create a dopamine response that makes them chemically addictive. At most, free sugars should be used as a sweetener in your tea—a half teaspoon or so. Even better, avoid them completely. You'll learn to enjoy your tea without the sugar. After a week, you won't miss it at all.

But why can't we just burn up sugar for energy in our muscles without it hovering in the bloodstream for hours after eating it and causing all these medical problems?

The answer was revealed in 1927 by Dr. J. Shirley Sweeney, who compared the effects of a high-carbohydrate diet to a high-fat diet on the body's ability to metabolize sugars.[14]

For a test period of forty-eight hours, he fed one group of healthy medical students a diet heavy in refined sugars: candy, pastry, sugar, syrup, and white bread, along with other high-carbohydrate whole foods, such as baked potatoes, bananas, rice, and oatmeal. Together, these foods (some unhealthy, some healthy, but all rich in carbohydrates) would have put lots of glucose into the bloodstream for the pancreas to handle by secreting insulin.

The other group of students was fed a diet based on high-fat foods including olive oil, butter, and mayonnaise made with egg yolk and 20 percent cream, with carbohydrates almost absent.

At the end of the forty-eight hours, both groups were given a standard "glucose tolerance test" commonly used to diagnose diabetes: The subjects drank a sweet liquid with seventy-five grams of glucose dissolved in it and, two hours later, blood sugar levels were measured to see how well the glucose load was handled. In people with adequate insulin production and function, the blood sugar should return to well below the 140 mg/dL range just two hours after swallowing the bolus of concentrated glucose. A number higher than that, from 140 to 199 mg/dL, puts one in the range of prediabetes, and over 200 mg/dL earns you an official diagnosis of diabetes.

The students who had been fed the high-carbohydrate diet, after forty-eight hours of their pancreas pumping out high levels of insulin to cope with the sugar overload and their cells metabolizing it, had no problem handling the test load of glucose. Within two hours of eating, the blood sugar of all those students had returned to nondiabetic levels, most well below the 120 mg/dL range.

On the other hand, the previously nondiabetic students who had been eating the high-fat diet all showed blood sugars in the plainly prediabetic range of 140 mg/dL or higher.

Clearly, it was the fat, not the sugar, that put these healthy medical students into the prediabetic range. (Don't worry about those long-dead 1927 test subjects, though: Within two days of resuming their normal, lower-fat diet, all the students had their blood sugar levels return to normal range—another early clue as to the reversibility of insulin resistance and type 2 diabetes.)

What was going on with these test subjects, and does it offer a lesson for us today?

We know this: Fat is an essential macronutrient that causes no problems when eaten in modest amounts in such whole plant foods as nuts, seeds, avocados, and olives. But when the Standard American Diet, laden with fatty meats, dairy products, and vegetable oils, repeatedly floods the tissues with heavy saturated fats and trans-fats, the lipid molecules begin to accumulate in muscle cells as intramyocellular lipid.

This is not a theoretical consideration. Here is what it looks like in muscle tissue, with the fat showing as black matter inside the muscle cells:

Fat in Muscle Tissue = Intramyocellular Lipid

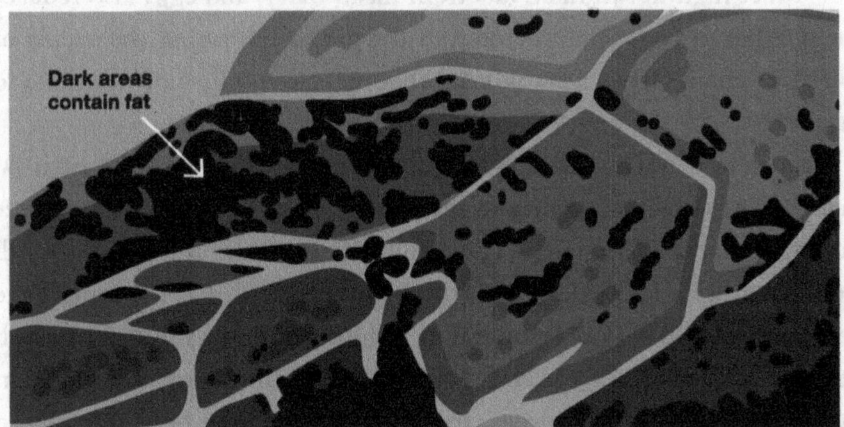

Insulin molecules chemically knock on the insulin receptor door, but nobody answers, because fats gum up the enzymatic gears. Consequently, glucose piles up in the bloodstream, creating the sugary mischief in blood vessel linings and the body's tissues for which diabetes is known. But it's important to remember: The high glucose levels in the blood are the *result* of the insulin resistance, not the cause. Fortunately, this is a reversible condition that can be turned around, believe it or not, often in mere days to weeks.

Simply put, if there are no other underlying medical causes (discussion of several to come), insulin resistance is brought on by eating too much fat. The fat chronically in the blood also exerts its sugar-elevating effects by another less direct, but still potent, mechanism, contributing to adipose tissue load inside the abdomen. You see, more than being just of cosmetic concern, a protruding abdomen is filled with visceral fat, which, in most obese people, releases a steady stream of inflammatory cytokines, such as interleukin-1 (IL-1) and interleukin-6 (IL-6), into the bloodstream. Along with their inflammation-stoking activities in many tissues, IL-1 and IL-6 also interfere with the function of the insulin receptors on the surface of the cell, further increasing insulin resistance.

A diet high in saturated fats from meat, dairy, and eggs also reduces the number of beneficial microbes in the gut, diminishing the supply of the short-chain fatty acids (SCFAs) that make the cells more sensitive to insulin.[15]

It's clear why Dr. Sweeney's healthy medical students fed a high-fat diet showed decreased ability to metabolize glucose, with resulting prediabetic numbers after forty-eight hours: Their insulin receptors were all clogged up with fat. Indeed, it is the high-fat diet that is a driving force behind most of the global tsunami of insulin resistance and diabetes that permeates so much of medical practice today. In the modern era, Dr. Sweeney's findings of fat-driven insulin resistance have been reproduced many times.[16] It is clearly today's high-fat diet that makes the jaws of insulin resistance—and eventual diabetes—open wide.

I was not taught this basic fact of nutrition in medical school. Nor, as far as I can discern, are most medical school students in America today being taught the dietary cause of type 2 diabetes, extraordinarily enough. When we list factors that can contribute to insulin resistance, medical ignorance of nutrition surely ranks near the top of the list.

Of course, there are other factors that can contribute to insulin resistance and its resulting high blood sugar levels.

Genetics certainly may play a role; we must always look for a family history to detect a genetic predisposition to the development of insulin resistance. Family history of diabetes or metabolic syndrome certainly increases the risk of an individual manifesting the disease. We must keep in mind, however, that we inherit not only our genes from our parents but also our eating habits. Surely, the diets we are fed in childhood, as well as our daily food choices that we flow through our cells with every meal, are strong determinants of which genes are activated in our cells and which are silenced through a process called *methylation*, wherein a small cluster of atoms (a carbon atom with three hydrogens) becomes attached to a gene on the DNA strand and keeps it from expressing its associated enzyme, thus "silencing" it.

Methylation is just one pathway by which our environment—especially the food we eat, whose molecules flow through every cell in our body after every meal—can influence how our genetic heritage is actually expressed, a process called *epigenetics*.

Our foods exert powerful epigenetic (gene-activating) influences over our cellular physiology, and that is certainly the case when it comes to metabolizing glucose.

And there are other factors at play beyond diet.

Physical inactivity contributes to the condition. How? As animals, we are meant to move during most of our day, and that movement requires that glucose be moved into the muscle cells to be metabolized for energy. As should be no surprise, sedentary lifestyles, in which powerful leg muscles sit quietly under computer desks for most of the day, contribute to higher sugar levels in the blood.

The **prolonged stress** that we inflict upon ourselves in just living this pressure-filled modern life presents another conspirator against normal blood sugar levels. Living in this state, hour after hour, day after day, can lead to the increased release of cortisol from our adrenal glands. This hormone, in turn, can increase blood sugar levels and contribute to insulin resistance.

Poor sleep quality and sleep disorders, such as sleep apnea, are also associated with increased insulin resistance.

Other, more rare, contributors to high glucose levels include the **hormonal imbalances** seen in conditions such as polycystic ovary syndrome (PCOS) and Cushing's syndrome that can lead to hormonal changes that reduce insulin sensitivity.

Certain **medications** can either create or exacerbate the problem: glucocorticoids (like hydrocortisone and prednisone), antipsychotics, and certain protease-inhibiting HIV treatments can promote insulin resistance.

Aging is also a factor. Our insulin receptors age along with the rest of us; their sensitivity tends to decrease with the years, making older adults more prone to insulin resistance.

Nutritional deficiencies, as well, may enter the equation. People with deficiencies in certain nutrients, such as magnesium and vitamin D, may be at higher risk for insulin resistance. In those cases, nutritional supplements can help. In the initial rounds of blood testing to track down the cause of the elevated blood sugars, checking the levels of 25(OH) vitamin D would likely be wise. Taking a multivitamin with supplemental vitamin D (approximately 2,000 IU or 50 mcg) per day and 200 mcg to 500 mcg of chromium can also boost insulin function.[17]

The most common cause of type 2 diabetes, nonetheless, remains an overly fatty diet. This fact should be screamingly obvious merely from the clear link between obesity and type 2 diabetes. Too much fat in the diet, especially when combined with refined sugars and flour products, makes you fat, and it also makes you diabetic. Ninety percent of type 2 diabetics are overweight or obese.[18] Fortunately, as Dr. Sweeney's students demonstrated, as long as one's pancreas can still produce adequate amounts of insulin, the resistance to the hormone and the resulting type 2 diabetes are eminently reversible conditions. Just as you can lose weight by reducing the percentage and type of fat in your diet, you can, at the same time and by the same method, reverse type 2 diabetes.

Doctors need to clearly and enthusiastically share this fact with their patients. It gives patients hope that they can truly be done with insulin shots, misguided carbo-phobic dietary restrictions, and living under the worry cloud of blindness, kidney failure, and amputation. Knowing that their type 2 diabetes is reversible, and that the process lies within their control via their daily food choices, empowers patients tremendously and should be discussed with vigor.

The reversibility of type 2 diabetes can be easily understood this way: Muscle and liver cells are always hungry for metabolizable molecules to burn in their mitochondrial furnaces. As the food stream and, thus, the bloodstream are freed of repeated surges of saturated fats, the liver and muscles will start shoveling into the mitochondria the energy-rich intramyocellular lipid accumulations already present in their cells. As the enzyme-clogging lipids are burned off, the insulin receptors start to function normally and healthy blood sugar levels return.

One successful approach to demonstrate the reversibility of type 2 diabetes was elegantly conducted by Dr. Neal Barnard and his research team. In 2009, they compared two cohorts, with one group of subjects consuming the (fairly low-carbohydrate) diet recommended by the American Diabetes Association, while the other nourished themselves on a low-fat vegan diet.[19] While there were improvements to the subjects' HgbA1c levels with both diets, the improvement was more than twice as great on the low-fat vegan diet. The low-fat vegan diet also produced three times as much reduction in total cholesterol and LDL cholesterol levels.

Reversing type 2 diabetes must involve diligent care from a doctor who carefully monitors the patient's medication. Deprescribing insulin and oral hypoglycemic agents like metformin requires a skilled hand.

On a healthy, high-fiber diet, the cellular cleanup and rebalancing that lead to type 2 diabetes reversal typically happen in a matter of days to weeks. As insulin receptors regain their function, the measured dosage of insulin that had previously been needed to keep blood sugar levels reasonable in a fat-choked metabolism may suddenly be far too high. In this state of unintentional insulin overdose, blood sugar levels can plummet to dangerously low levels, injuring brain cells as they do.

Both doctor and patient must stand ready to reduce dosages of insulin and other hypoglycemic medications rapidly, but not too abruptly. Like many things in medicine, there is a bit of an art to deprescribing insulin and oral hypoglycemic agents such as metformin without endangering the patient. I recommend to my medical colleagues to take guidance from the adage, "better too sweet than sour." That is, we can walk around for hours with a high blood sugar, well over 200 mg/dL, but a blood sugar of less than 30 mg/dL held for any significant time may well induce a seizure or even coma and can do serious long-term damage to the brain. When regaining consciousness after such a prolonged hypoglycemic blackout, we would likely suffer some degree of impairment of cognitive function.

Therefore, the person weaning off insulin should check their blood sugar at least four times a day: upon waking up, before going to sleep, and two hours before and after at least one meal of the day, preferably the meal with the most starch. If the fasting glucose numbers have held between 80 and 130 mg/dL, and the value two hours after eating is less than 180 mg/dL, the person can reduce the units of insulin by 10 to 20 percent—under the watchful eye and assent of their primary care provider. So, a patient who had been taking thirty units of long-acting insulin in the morning could reduce it by three to six units every few days, as described. After a few days, if the fasting and two-hour post-meal glucose numbers are holding steady as above, the insulin dosage may be knocked down another 10 to 20 percent. The patient may continue in this manner until the ten-unit-per-day dosage is reached; at that point, the insulin can be stopped altogether, with careful monitoring to see if the blood sugar levels remain healthfully low. (If the numbers stay stubbornly high, then a search for other medical causes, such as hidden infection or type 1.5 diabetes—an autoimmune condition in adults characterized by antibodies attacking the insulin-producing beta cells in the pancreas—should be conducted.)

For the person taking metformin or other hypoglycemic agents, once the insulin has been stopped and the glucose measurements remain in the aforementioned limits for fasting and post-eating times, the dose of the oral agent can be reduced by half, and then, after five to seven days, if blood sugars stay acceptable, stopped altogether. If there are significant symptoms of low blood sugar, and/or hypoglycemic blood values (below 70 mg/dL), the oral agents should be stopped immediately. Wearing a continuous glucose monitor (CGM) would be extremely valuable for patients during this phase of insulin adjustments. In this way, both patient and practitioner can track the realities of the blood sugar levels.

At all times during this process, both patient and practitioner must remain vigilant for signs of too low a blood sugar (hypoglycemia) manifesting as headache, sweating, lightheadedness, and/or rapid pulse. If, as measured by finger stick or, ideally, on their CGM, the person's blood sugar level remains low and falling, or if the person is symptomatic or even suspects they may become so, they should immediately ingest some sugar in some form—a hard candy, a glass of fruit juice, or a glucose tablet available at any pharmacy, which should be carried by everyone who uses insulin.

Why, you may wonder, do we hear proponents of meat-heavy diets, like the Paleo and keto diets, report dramatically lower blood sugars with their fat-heavy food plan? Aren't their insulin receptors all clogged up from all the fat they eat?

Yes, they certainly are, but, since they eat so little sugar in their rabidly anti-carb diet, which consists of mostly just fat and protein (usually from animal foods), along with very-low-glycemic vegetables, they put almost no glucose in their bloodstream. Their glucose levels stay low in their blood not because they are not insulin resistant—as they most likely are—but simply because they just never eat the stuff.

If the left turn signal in your car is broken, one solution would be to have it fixed. The other solution—the keto solution, if you will—would be to never make a left turn again. Make enough right turns, they would argue, and you can get wherever you want to go. Theoretically, it's doable, but which approach strikes you as more sustainable?

Unfortunately, if those practicing a keto diet *do* eat any glucose-containing foods (*gasp!*), their fat-clogged insulin receptors will predictably shoot their blood glucose to high levels, prompting the keto proponents to gleefully proclaim, "See! I told you those bad ol' carbs will skyrocket your blood sugar! Avoid them at all costs!"

But what are we looking at here? Is this not a physiologic parlor trick? We make ourselves insulin resistant with all the fat in the diet and then watch a dollop of glucose cause elevated blood sugar levels. That is no reason to avoid our mitochondria's favorite fuel, glucose; rather, it is an argument to avoid high-fat diets and to eat whole plant foods whose lipids and carbohydrates alike are delivered with plenty of fiber that slows down their absorption, as well as with vitamins and minerals that will aid in their digestion and metabolism.

As one adopts the high-fiber, WPF eating style, type 2 diabetes automatically begins to resolve via the following mechanisms:

1. Sensitivity to insulin improves as intramyocellular lipid is metabolized.
2. The higher fiber intake slows absorption of glucose into the bloodstream.
3. The weight loss that naturally occurs from the lower calorie density of whole plant foods reduces visceral fat and its inflammatory cytokine production, both of which interfere with insulin receptor function.
4. Very importantly, abundant antioxidant molecules in the plant-rich food stream will protect the beta cells from the oxidative damage that eventually leads to beta cell loss and, thus, permanent need for exogenous insulin.

Therefore, I would advise all physicians who treat type 2 diabetes to consider that helping your patient transition to a low-fat, whole-food, plant-based food stream should be the essential first step in reversing their condition. The other pillars of lifestyle medicine—a daily walk in the sunshine, adequate sleep, minimized stress level, involvement in community and/or family, and avoidance of toxic substances (and relationships!)—play vital roles in not only normalizing blood sugar levels but also helping a fellow human to regain their health.

Prevention and Reversal of Hypertension

We have examined the mechanisms by which a change from a fatty Western diet of animal foods to a whole plant food diet may prevent and reverse cardiovascular disease and type 2 diabetes. Common sense might give you an inkling that the diet that is right for preventing and reversing these modern plagues might prove beneficial for all manner of other health concerns, and indeed that is the case with hypertension.

The definition of hypertension has been a moving target in the United States. The current definition has been reduced to a systolic blood pressure (SBP) of 130 mm Hg or greater and/or a diastolic blood pressure (DBP) of 80 mm Hg or greater. Before 2017, hypertension had been defined as commencing at a reading of 140/90 for those under age sixty-five, and 150/80 for those sixty-five and up. What happened to bring about this revision to what doctors should view, and treat, as hypertension?

One explanation derives from a charitable view of our medical system: Rigorous, objective science has determined that a blood pressure of 130/80, which used to be considered acceptable, may actually have deleterious effects on human health. So in the interest of our patients' health, we doctors must begin to treat our patients who hover in that range, with the aim of lowering their blood pressure to healthier levels.

The other explanation is more cynical: By defining hypertension down, in one fell swoop the medical system has added many millions more people to the pool of those who are candidates for beta-blockers and other pharmaceuticals. Big Pharma, it could be argued, must be thrilled with the new definition of hypertension and must have lobbied for it.

I may not win many friends by saying this, but I believe that both explanations may be true. I see no reason to consider them mutually exclusive.

Here again, though, an understanding of nutrition is key. For a patient with blood pressure in the previously-normal-but-suddenly-concerning neighborhood of 130/80, there is no reason to jump to a pharmaceutical remedy, which will frequently be accompanied by side effects. Nutritional therapy should be attempted first. In the well-known EPIC-Oxford study,[20] the blood pressure of some eleven thousand British citizens, divided into vegans, vegetarians, pescatarians, and meat eaters, was analyzed. The vegans fared the best, with the lowest blood pressure. The meat eaters had the worst scores, with the vegetarians and pescatarians in the middle range. More than twenty years ago, a study was conducted on the DASH ("Dietary Approaches to Stop Hypertension") diet, which is not a vegan diet but is high in fruits, vegetables, and whole grains and relatively low in animal products. That less-than-optimal but plant-strong diet substantially reduced blood pressure.[21]

A meta-analysis of some thirty-nine blood pressure studies published in *Current Hypertension Reports* in 2023 concluded that "The overwhelming majority of intervention studies demonstrate that plant-based diets result in lower blood pressure readings when compared to diets that are based on animal products . . . The data discussed in this systematic review allow us to conclude that plant-based diets are associated with lower blood pressure and overall better health outcomes (namely, on the cardiovascular system) when compared to animal-based diets."[22]

The meta-analysis of thirty-nine studies proposed some mechanisms to explain the beneficial effects of a plant-based diet on blood pressure. One was the notion that ascorbic acid (vitamin C) stimulates nitric oxide production; nitric oxide plays a crucial role in vasodilation, the widening of our blood vessels. Another suggested mechanism: The potassium in such foods as green leafy vegetables, bananas, and potatoes contributes to natriuresis, the process leading to the excretion of sodium in the urine. The paper also theorized that vasodilation may be augmented by polyphenols and other antioxidant-rich compounds in plant foods.

I would expect that all these proposed mechanisms have validity, and I would add one more: A diet rich in plant foods will generally be lower in animal-based foods. And the saturated fat and cholesterol in animal-based foods build up plaque in the arteries, stiffening and narrowing them, raising peripheral resistance, and consequently raising blood pressure.

Unsurprisingly, therefore, the medical literature overwhelmingly supports the thesis that plant-rich diets lower blood pressure. Of course, we know that nutritional studies often contradict each other; it seems that you can find a study, if you look hard enough, to support virtually any nutritional proposition. In my review of the literature, I did find one single study that proposed a blood-pressure-lowering effect to beef consumption.[23] That study, you won't be shocked to learn, was funded by the Beef Checkoff program.

To any objective reader of the voluminous evidence, the beneficial effect of a plant-based diet on blood pressure is hard to dispute. How important is blood pressure to your well-being? A consistent high blood pressure reading is the red "check engine light" of health. It tells you that any number of things may go wrong soon, and you may be in serious danger. As far as I know, there isn't a quack alive who promotes high blood pressure as a desirable state. It is settled science that high blood pressure can lead to stroke, heart disease, kidney damage, vision loss, peripheral artery disease, brain damage, and more—and manage to do so painlessly. This is why it is known as *the silent killer.*

If a physician has no choice but to control a patient's blood pressure with medications, then that must be done. But pharmaceutical remedies—and there's a wide array of choices for hypertension—present their own risks. Beta-blockers may bring on arrhythmia, nausea, sexual dysfunction, and diarrhea. Diuretics can cause headache, urinary frequency, fatigue, gout, low electrolytes, dehydration, and even hypovolemia (a dangerous condition of low blood plasma). Calcium-channel blockers may result in fatigue, dizziness, constipation, and peripheral edema. Vasodilators may bring on irregular heartbeat, nausea, fever, dizziness, and muscle pain. ACE inhibitors can bring on dry cough, hypotension, edema, jaundice, and hyperkalemia (too much potassium in the blood).

There are no such side effects from leafy greens and other vegetables, whole grains, fruits, and legumes.

Chapter Four

UNDERSTANDING NUTRITIONAL THERAPY, PART TWO

Best Strategies for Gastrointestinal Disorders, Fatty Liver Disease, Alzheimer's Disease, Covid-19, ALS, and Alpha-Gal Syndrome

Let us look now at some other common diseases afflicting our population. For some of these, we can promise prevention and even reversal through diet therapy. For others, there is reason to believe that they can be prevented through diet, or that diet can at least reduce one's chances of developing the disease, but there can be no promise of reversal. For yet others, the benefit of diet does not concern prevention or reversal but rather easing the severity of the symptoms.

Prevention and Reversal of Gastrointestinal Disorders

Each of the many times I have pulled a chart out of the holder on the exam room door, and the nurse has written on it "abdominal pain," I have felt my own guts tighten a bit inside. Pain in the abdomen is one of the great diagnostic challenges in medicine. The physician's anxiety in treating abdominal pain stems from the very real fear of misdiagnosis. Standing at the side of such a patient, physicians must therefore use all their clinical cunning to divine what malevolent forces may be causing visceral chaos within that sacrosanct space of the abdominal cavity. This is an archetypal medical act, one that I have always taken seriously.

A good deal of information offers itself to the physician's eyes and ears as the bedside is approached. Is the patient lying comfortably on the gurney or writhing in pain? Does the patient sit up when I approach? If they do, it is a likely sign that no organ is inflamed within. Or does the person lie quietly, with brow furrowed and their hands caressing a particular part of their belly? Then, depending upon the location of the pain, which the person is often able to pinpoint with precision, infected tissue is likely present. Here in the West, the most likely site will be in the appendix, gallbladder, or—as with diverticulitis—the intestinal wall.

Is the patient, by contrast, writhing in agony on the bed, unable to lie quietly, and, when asked to locate the pain, indicates vaguely "all over their belly?" Then this suggests the clinical picture of a bowel obstruction. A tumor (a benign or malignant mass), a cancer invading the gut wall, or a fibrous adhesion is almost surely present, with a distended, contracting colon contorting as it tries to push a mass of stool past the site of obstruction. Here, the remedy usually requires the surgeon's blade and, in the best of scenarios, a capable general surgeon would be immediately summoned and forthwith appear on the scene. If she or he concurs with the diagnosis after appropriate testing, the patient would be transported to the operating room where, under anesthesia, the pathology would be excised and harmony surgically restored within the peritoneum.

Thankfully, the bellies that physicians confront most often in their office practice are not "acute abdomens." Far more frequently, the problem is a chronic one, mostly of disordered bowel function: constipation, impacted stool, stools too hard, diarrhea, stools too loose, painful evacuations, blood in the stool, mucus in the stool, and intestinal gas and bloating.

Most of my primary care colleagues traditionally confront many of these complaints and symptoms as individual foes to be vanquished. Attending to a patient presenting with gas, distention, abdominal cramps, and loose stools—the classic irritable bowel syndrome (IBS)—there may be a few blind stabs at dietary manipulations. "Don't eat beans," the patient might be told, "they give you gas." If the complaint seems sufficiently serious or has endured for some time, this minimal dietary advice will likely be quickly followed by a referral to a gastroenterologist. Often, an additional impetus for the referral is a subconscious belief in the back of the doctor's mind that "this is all in the patient's head"—implying there is some deep, psychological problem that the patient is playing out by focusing on abdominal complaints. Even a physician convinced of the reality of the patient's pain might feel that its equally real cause is psychological stress. Either way, the referral to the gastroenterologist provides a face-saving escape valve for the primary care physician who doesn't want to play psychiatrist, while still raising hope in the patient's mind for relief of their symptoms.

Once in the office of the GI specialist, who is always fearful of missing an early (or advanced) bowel cancer, the patient generally finds that the doctor recommends inspecting the large intestine with a scope procedure. This consists of inserting one of the most ingenious and useful tools invented in the last decades: the colonoscope. This small, well-lubricated, flexible tube, filled with bendable optical fibers, permits the health of the colon wall to be visually inspected. If a suspicious area is noted by the operator, biopsy samples of the lining can be taken and sent to the pathologist. A full colonoscopy may be indicated in order to remove precancerous polyps, identify sites of bleeding, or inspect the ileocecal valve. However, a colonoscopy is never a comfortable procedure—nor, for those who must pay, is it inexpensive, and it carries a small but serious risk of setting off bleeding or creating a perforation high in the colon that would require emergency surgery to repair. I feel strongly that a colonoscopy should thus be reserved for individuals with specific medical issues that require that procedure (bleeding, unexplained pain, family history of colon cancer) rather than using it for repeatedly screening the general public. Having said that, there is a better case to be made for colonoscopy screenings for those eating the Standard American Diet than for those on the WPF diet, who are not regularly smearing their colons with carcinogens. Patients should discuss with their doctor whether a sigmoidoscopy—a less uncomfortable procedure, which visualizes only the lower two feet of the colon, but does includes the S-shaped, "sigmoid" colon, where most cancers and inflammatory conditions are found—might be indicated, either to diagnose a condition or as a screening tool. Those patients who don't want to undergo either the colonoscopy or the sigmoidoscopy also have the pain-free option of checking their stool for occult blood every two years.

Do these often-uncomfortable testing procedures yield definitive pathologies and point the way to effective treatment? Alas, when it comes to our patient with the cramps, gas, and bloating after meals, the scope procedures almost always find that all looks "essentially normal" in the intestinal wall. A diagnosis of IBS is made and nary a thought given to the possible effects that their patient's diet might be having upon the health and function of their gut. At this point, the gastroenterologist is reduced to controlling symptoms: the gas, pain, bloating, diarrhea, constipation, and inflammation that plague the patient. And, thanks to the development of ever more potent pharmaceuticals, physicians have an increasingly powerful armamentarium to use for that job—bringing along with it an equally daunting array of side effects that they tell themselves they can wrestle with later.

More and more commonly, the patient is informed that their only hope to live a normal life is to take regular injections of expensive, powerful drugs that inhibit their immune systems and may open them up to lethal infections and cancers. The possibility of a wholesale change in diet rarely enters the discussion.

This disregard of diet amounts to a stunning blind spot in the minds of too many gastroenterologists. Of all the medical specialties, one would think that the physicians whose daily medical practices focus on the health and function of the digestive system would at least recognize and consider the powerful effects—positive or negative—that the food stream flowing through thirty miraculous feet of biological tubing exerts on the health and function of the gut wall, and, indeed, the entire body.

It would seem to take a major effort of will to ignore or overlook the mechanisms that, if given a moment's thought, would loom large as significant factors in the disease doctors strive to treat.

The quality of our food stream—what it contains and what it doesn't—acts like an orchestra conductor who, with a wave of her hands, brings up the woodwinds and tones down the brass. The amounts of sugars, proteins, fats, and fibers in the food stream will bring up the populations of certain microbes, as others recede due to lack of their favored nutrients. The "good guy" and the "bad guy" microbes already live within us; it is the food stream we choose to flow through our gut that will determine if the overall balance becomes benevolent or disruptive.

The animal-food-rich, fatty Western diet militates daily against gut health. The vaunted proteins in meat and dairy products are heavy with amino acids like taurine, cysteine, and cystine that contain an atom of sulfur. The bacteria that these animal-based foods foster will metabolize those amino acids, and, in doing so, liberate molecules of hydrogen sulfide gas (H2S), which diffuses into nearby intestinal cells. In this watery milieu, the H2S generates sulfurous acid, a potent irritant to all cells and tissues, including the nearby gut wall. Since meat and dairy are usually eaten daily by most Westerners, the almost constant presence of these acid-generating substances will, in many people, kindle inflammation. It often manifests first as the cramps, gas, and bloating of IBS, and, in some unfortunate folks, progresses to the pain and bloody diarrhea of inflammatory bowel disease (IBD). This condition is often subdivided into ulcerative colitis in the large bowel and the devastating Crohn's disease, which usually targets the wall of the small intestine.

However defined, these diseases wreck people's lives. Patients are left feeling like helpless victims, seemingly at the mercy of a mutinous digestive system. They view their gut as a demon in their belly that capriciously, often diabolically, sends them scurrying for the nearest toilet, making enjoying a two-hour movie a virtual impossibility and transforming air travel into a nightmare. They feel trapped by a disease that inflicts pain, fatigue, and social disruption upon them, to which they can respond only with food restriction or medication that is often expensive and not always effective.

Most ominously, the constant exposure of the colon wall cells to cancer-causing chemicals—the H2S-generated acids, the cancer-promoting degradation products of bile ("secondary bile acids") that the stool now contains (evoked by the higher fat content of the animal foods consumed), as well as the outright carcinogens inevitably generated by the cooking of meat that repeatedly smears on the same part of the colon wall—may finally blossom forth as a GI cancer, the second most common cause of cancer death in both men and women.

Beyond that, the food stream dictated by the standard food choices made by most Americans—high in animal foods, high in fat, high in processed foods and sugar—reliably contains a platoon of molecular marauders that assault the normal structure and function of the intestinal lining in many ways.

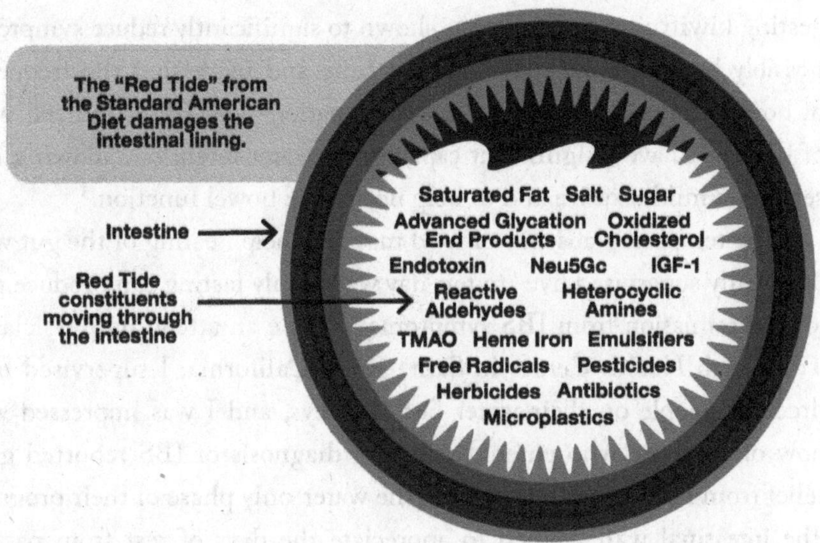

For example, in IBS, characterized by cramps, gas, bloating, diarrhea, or constipation, the bowels may indeed be irritable about what is being smeared upon their inner membranes every few hours. Eliminating gluten, dairy, meat, wheat, soy, and eggs has produced significant improvements in IBS symptoms; this is my recommended first step in letting the bowels regain their normal function.

If elimination of the above products does not result in a significant improvement, the IBS sufferer may benefit from eliminating foods with a collection of sugars widely known as *FODMAPs* (fermentable oligosaccharides, disaccharides, monosaccharides, and polyols). These foods include garlic, onion, wheat, rye, barley, leek, asparagus, chicory, artichoke, and some legumes, such as lentils, chickpeas, and kidney beans. If relief is obtained by this elimination trial for several weeks, FODMAP-containing foods are then reintroduced in a controlled manner, per the protocol developed by nutrition researchers at Australia's Monash University.[1]

Some patients have also reported dramatic symptom relief with the use of probiotic products containing multiple strains of bifidobacteria.

IBS is certainly a condition for which food can serve as medicine. Ingesting kiwifruit twice daily has shown to significantly reduce symptoms, possibly by shortening colon transit time and increasing the frequency of bowel emptying in those with constipation-type IBS.[2] The cell walls of kiwifruit have a significant capacity for water retention, allowing it to serve as a mild laxative and to help normalize bowel function.[3]

The temporary absence of food may also help healing of the gut wall. Medically supervised five- to ten-day water-only fasting can produce prolonged remission from IBS symptoms.[4] While an attending physician at TrueNorth Health Center in Santa Rosa, California, I supervised hundreds of people on their water fast journeys, and I was impressed with how often those who entered with the diagnosis of IBS reported great relief from their symptoms during the water-only phase of their program. The intestinal wall seemed to appreciate the days of rest from passing irritating food masses; this therapy allowed inflammation to subside, the microbiome to rebalance, and the digestive system to regain the rhythms of its function. Be aware: *Extended water fasts (longer than forty-eight hours) must always be medically supervised.*

Crohn's disease, a vicious autoimmune condition featuring an aggressive inflammatory process that is unleashed in the wall of the small intestine and that can burrow into neighboring structures, such as the bladder, vagina, or colon, is made clinically worse by numerous components in food. The animal tissue in meat and fish inevitably contains remnants of blood that degrade into carbon monoxide, aldehydes, carcinogens, and other toxic molecules produced when the meat is cooked, as well as the pro-inflammatory arachidonic acid that is present in all animal muscle. This rogues' gallery of problematic molecules combine to stoke the quality-of-life-destroying, inflammatory fires of Crohn's disease.

How does it all start? The process may be initiated when the gut's inner, mucosal lining is injured from agents in food, including commonly used food ingredients such as emulsifiers—for example: polysorbate 80, carboxymethylcellulose (CMC), lecithins, mono- and diglycerides, guar gum and xanthan gum, propylene glycol alginate, and, possibly, carrageenan, a seaweed derivative. These substances give ice cream and candy bars their pleasant mouth feel, but they also may loosen the tight junctions between cells, which would increase the gut wall's permeability to toxic substances from food and microbes and also thin the mucus layer that lines our intestinal tract.[5, 6] Reducing the effectiveness of this mucus layer, even partially, could allow molecules such as inflammation-inciting endotoxins to enter the bloodstream and taint tissues around the body. But more worrisome, the now leakier gut allows pathogenic strains of *E. coli*, *Mycobacterium avium subspecies paratuberculosis*, and other gut bacteria to burrow deep into the intestinal wall where reactive lymphocytes reside. There, like saboteurs deep behind enemy lines who stumble onto an ammunition depot, they set off a vicious firefight, igniting the smoldering inflammation that can burn for weeks if untreated, causing unremitting pain, diarrhea, and bleeding. Over time, this may chemically burn holes through the gut wall. These excavations can then burrow into nearby vital organs, with dreadful results. A permanent channel between the small intestine and the bladder (an enterovesical fistula) would have the person passing stool in their urinary stream.

Diets low in fiber put patients at risk for Crohn's disease, possibly from lack of butyrate production needed to restore gut wall integrity. (Butyrate is a short-chain fatty acid linked to many health benefits.) Once Crohn's disease is established and active, the patient must avoid raw, poorly chewed fiber in salads and crudités. Rather, foods like blended squash, rice congee, or melon chunks provide fiber in a softer, more benevolent form that can be soothing for the gut wall. Also, since yeast products, including bread and beer, have long been shown to be hazardous for people with Crohn's disease, they are also best avoided to minimize flare-ups of symptoms.

Certainly, the best strategy remains avoiding consumption of the foods that create these insults to our digestive systems in the first place. Taking advantage of the medicinal qualities of some foods can also help: Components found in broccoli and plantain can inhibit pathogenic microbes from invading the deeper tissues.[7] Spices like clove, oregano, thyme, cinnamon, and cumin possess antifungal and antibacterial properties that can help prevent gastrointestinal disorders arising from food spoilage.[8] Fruits such as black currants, grapes, and cranberries, and their extracts, have similar protective properties.[9]

As with virtually all health issues, a pattern emerges: Animal foods, in general, create inflammation and foster development of disease; plant foods have protective and anti-inflammatory properties.

In fact, even a "semi-vegetarian" diet, far inferior to a diet I would personally recommend, in which people consume a fiber-rich, plant-based diet on a daily basis, while eating only a small portion of fish weekly and a half portion of other meat but twice a month, with small quantities of eggs and dairy also regrettably included, has been shown to keep Crohn's disease in remission for years.[10] It is remarkable to see this fearsome malady—that turns sections of the inside of the small intestine into a fiery, swollen, bleeding tube—recede under the influence of a healing, plant-based diet, with the small intestine reverting to its pink, healthy state, once again digesting normally and absorbing vital nutrients from food.

In ulcerative colitis, where the wall of the large intestine is inflamed and bleeding, major culprits are the acidic byproducts, such as hydrogen sulfide, sulfur dioxide, and thiocyanate, among others, that are produced from the sulfur-containing amino acids that abound in eggs, milk, pork, chicken, and fish. Avoiding these foods by consuming a whole-food, plant-based diet predictably produces significant improvements in this dreadful condition.

As in Crohn's disease, the bleeding, pockmarked colon wall stands eminently capable of healing itself and restoring normal structure and function, if given a soothing, high-fiber diet with little or, better, none of the inflammatory animal foods mentioned above. Patients who are educated about the healing effect of a whole plant food diet and who implement such a food program usually achieve dramatic improvements of their symptoms and become among the most grateful any physician will ever encounter in their practice.

In treating any variety of inflammatory bowel disease, whether Crohn's disease or ulcerative colitis, potent, anti-inflammatory medications must often be used. These include corticosteroids or one of the newer "biologic" agents that inhibit components of the inflammatory process. I have no quarrel with the use of these agents, though I would hope they would be used in the lowest dose to achieve remission of symptoms.

As any physician who, in support of suffering patients, has grappled with these tenacious diseases knows, the trick is how to get the patient off these suppressive medications without precipitating a flare-up of the inflammation. That is where a healing diet comes in.

The strategy that has worked so often for me and my nutrition-aware colleagues is to keep the patient on a low dose of prednisone or other inflammation-modifying agent (after tapering down from the original therapeutic dose) for as many weeks as needed to fully suppress their inflammatory symptoms. During this time, their now plant-based food stream (if necessary, low in FODMAP-containing foods), allows the gut wall to heal and reconstitute itself. It will also foster growth of a newer, more benign population of microbes that will colonize the gut surface. Then, when symptoms have receded to negligible levels, the steroids and other drugs are finally tapered off and stopped. Usually, much to the delight of both doctor and patient, the feared flare-up does not occur.

Regrettably, in standard medical practice today, the dietary patterns that can clearly play key roles in the prevention and reversal of these fearsome diseases are virtually never mentioned to the patient. In this way, the afflicted sufferer is denied the safest, most natural, most affordable, and lowest-risk strategies to free themselves of these diseases.

When I broach the subject of diet with GI colleagues, they generally shake their head and offer the following canards as to why the patient's diet has little or no place within their diagnostic or treatment paradigms:

"Food has no effect on these diseases."

"There never have been any studies that prove that food has any effect on (insert a GI disease here)."

"Diet has too many variables to consider its effect."

"Food is a cultural issue. It's not my place to tell someone from Mexico or India what they should be eating."

"People are never going to change what they eat."

"I've never had any training in nutrition—it's not my field, and I wouldn't know what to tell these people to eat."

"I don't have time to do nutritional counseling, and I don't get paid for doing it!"

In these words, I hear the clanging of the mental bars of the conceptual prisons these doctors have constructed for themselves and impose upon their patients, from whom they ultimately withhold strategies for true healing of their painful digestive scourges. Tragically, these doctors also deprive themselves of the deep satisfaction of seeing their chronically ill patients regain the treasured, warm glow of health.

Perhaps nowhere are the bars of the mental cages thickest as in those guarding the etiology of cancer of the colon. I am sure that most of my medical colleagues willingly accept the cause-and-effect mechanism demonstrated in the gruesome exercise in carcinogenesis we all learned about in pathology class. In this sad setup, a carcinogen, such as the benzo(a)pyrene found in cigarette smoke and cooked meats, is repeatedly rubbed on the skin of some poor, living creature, perhaps the ears of a rabbit. After weeks of these applications on the same spot of skin, an invasive, ulcerating, squamous cell carcinoma arises and proceeds to invade and destroy the surrounding tissue, and eventually, the rabbit itself.

None of the gastroenterologists I know have any problem with accepting the fact that repeated applications of a carcinogen to the same spot of tissue can induce an aggressive cancer. Yet they remain oblivious to the fact that the food stream that currently constitutes the Standard

American Diet remains redolent with known carcinogens and carcinogen-promoting agents, such as:

- Heterocyclic amines (HCAs) and polycyclic aromatic hydrocarbons (PAHs), such as benzo(a)pyrene, generated by cooking meat—charcoal grilling and barbecuing are the most prolific benzo(a)pyrene-generating cooking methods
- Nitrosamines from the nitrates used to preserve meats
- Saturated fats and cholesterol, which promote extra bile flow that bacteria convert to carcinogenic secondary bile acids
- Heme iron (derived from animal products only), which can promote the formation of cancer-causing N-nitroso compounds, as well as contribute to oxidative stress and inflammation in the colon, further increasing cancer risk
- Trimethylamine N-oxide (TMAO), produced from the metabolism of choline, lecithin, and carnitine (found in red meat, eggs, and dairy), which promotes inflammation, atherosclerosis, and cancer, including colon cancer
- Advanced glycation end products (AGEs), found in baked and fried carbohydrate-rich foods such as donuts and potato chips as well as in pasteurized dairy and cooked meat, which contribute to cancer-promoting oxidative stress and inflammation

Of course, the deleterious effects of the cancer-fanning agents named above are magnified by the low fiber content of the Western diet that allows the carcinogen-laden fecal masses to move extra slowly through the colon. This allows extra-long exposure times for the chemical saboteurs to rub against the colon wall tissues and incite malignant changes.

Finally, the saturated fats in the diet promote insulin resistance in the tissues, causing the pancreas to send extra amounts of insulin into the blood. Insulin promotes cell proliferation and cancer growth.[11]

One would think that any experienced medical practitioner who did not sleep through pathology class would see the similarities in the two carcinogen-slathering scenarios. Yet once again, the effects of food upon the body seem to be off-limits in this hallowed specialty, as well as most of the others. Has medicine divorced itself from science?

Studies of populations with differing diets do, indeed, show differing colon cancer risk. In the Adventist Health Study, the vegans had a 16 percent lower risk of colon cancer than people eating a meat-based diet. And people eating a mostly vegan diet with occasional fish ("pescatarians") had a 43 percent lower risk.[12]

It's simply logical that a significant reduction in colon cancer risk would be expected in a diet of whole plant foods (fruits, vegetables, whole grains, legumes, nuts, and seeds), given the higher intake of fiber, antioxidants, and phytonutrients. A diet high in fiber will promote healthy bowel movements, reducing the time the colon is exposed to potential carcinogens.

But why only a 16 percent reduction in risk for the vegans? And what's with the fish eaters enjoying a 43 percent reduction? Ah, herein lies exposed the Achilles' heel of nutritional studies. In recruiting subjects for these studies, people are asked to characterize their eating practices at the time of recruitment. That is, a person who had been eating flesh and dairy foods all life long, until seeing, a week earlier, the movie *Earthlings*—a powerful look at slaughterhouses and cruelty to farmed animals—and swearing off all animal products on the spot, could honestly check the box marked "vegan." At around the same time, a polyp in their colon that had been simmering with carcinogens and inflammatory compounds for months could finally cross the line into malignant growth. As it announces its presence three years later with bright red blood seen in the stools, the event will be chalked up in the study as "occurring in a vegan," when the seeds were actually sown in the dark, fleshy fecal stream that colon wall had been subjected to during many earlier non-vegan years.

Most people recruited into studies like EPIC-Oxford or the Adventist

Health Study made that contribution to science (yes, subjects of studies deserve credit) later in their lives. Very few subjects were raised as vegans since birth. Even if that rare person did show up in the study pool, their history as a distinct type of vegan would not be tracked, so they would remain unrecognized and, tragically, understudied.

I feel this is a great missed opportunity. People who have been raised as vegans since birth are unique human beings, in their biochemistry, their physiology, their microbiome, and probably even their brain functioning. Their actual dietary practices, along with their susceptibility to various diseases and their eventual cause of demise, should be of great interest to all of us. A registry to track vegans since birth should be started, to see what happens to these people, medically, over the long term. My anecdotal experience of several such people would lead me to predict a promising outcome.

So, hidden in that "16 percent reduction in risk" in the vegan population lives a lifetime of disease-generating dietary choices that make such population studies like these "low quality" in trying to tease out the effects of specific dietary styles over the long term. Similarly, regarding the "43 percent reduction of risk" in people who consume fish, one must ask: "How often do they consume the fish? Once a month? Once a week? What kind of fish? How is it prepared?" (The study defined the pesco-vegetarians as eating fish "one or more times a month.") There could be a variety of explanations for the apparent reduction. Are these fish-eating people more generally health conscious? Had they stuck to a relatively healthy, high-fiber, mostly-plant-based-with-occasional-fish diet, free of red meat and chicken and dairy, for years? Was the lower cancer risk due to the vegetables, with the fish intake bordering on irrelevant? Or even if, as the study's authors speculated, the pesco-vegetarians may have benefited from the long-chain omega-3 fatty acids in fish, might the same salutary effect have been achieved if the vegan cohort had obtained their omega-3 fatty acids from walnuts, hempseeds, and flaxseeds?

There are many variables that could have been in play here, but given the nutritional hazards of eating fish today—the mercury, pesticides, dioxins, microplastics, estrogen mimics, neurotoxins, and more—one can hardly conclude that adding fish to a plant-based diet constitutes a move in the direction of health.

For me, the clincher in the diet-cancer link was demonstrated in a discerning study conducted on a group of African Americans, who were compared with an equal number of Africans in rural South Africa. As background for this study, consider that the incidence of colon cancer has been skyrocketing among the African American population for the past several decades. The incidence of colon cancer in African Americans is ten times higher than in rural Africans.[13]

The reason for this difference is thought to be the quality of the diet of each group. American Blacks have, over the past decades, become prime consumers of the fast-food diet so prevalent in urban America: a deadly, low-fiber, overly processed food stream laden with cooked animal muscle, fried potatoes and onions, refined sugars and oils, and artificial colors, flavorings, and preservatives. The rural South Africans, on the other hand, largely adhered to their traditional diets, heavy with root vegetables, whole grains, legumes, and greens. Meat intake in this group was minimal in both quantity and frequency.

The study design was quite elegant. A colonoscopy examination was done on each participant, with the health of the colon assessed regarding inflammation and the presence of precancerous polyps. A small snip (biopsy) of colon lining was taken from each patient and sent to the pathologist to look for signs of inflammation that might promote cancer growth. The results, to me, spoke volumes.

The colonoscopies on the Western-diet group revealed signs of colons in trouble—polyps, diverticula, hemorrhoids—and their biopsies showed significant inflammation, with many white blood cells along with precancerous cell division evident. The rural South Africans exhibited colons that were much healthier, with almost no polyps or other colon problems and only minimal numbers of inflammatory cells on biopsy.

At that point, their diets were switched to their culinary and cultural opposites: the African Americans were given, essentially, an African-style, whole-food, plant-based diet, heavy with grains, beans, legumes, and vegetables, with only minimal amounts of meat, while the rural South Africans got to experience the glories of Western-style Egg McMuffin breakfasts, burgers-and-fries lunches, and dinners of meatloaf and white rice.

After two weeks on these "opposite" diets, a repeat colonoscopy and biopsy were performed on each patient. To my not-great surprise, the biopsies showed just the changes expected by such food streams: The rural South African biopsies showed the ravages of the repeated, Toxic Red Tide meals, with markedly increased inflammatory cell numbers and precancerous cell proliferation evident in each person, while after two weeks of the veggie-heavy, minimal-meat diet, the African American colon biopsies showed far less inflammation and exhibited a restoration of normal, noncancerous architecture. The healing tendency was unmistakable.

My only reservation about this elegant study: Was it perhaps cruel to the rural South Africans to expose them to the Western diet for two weeks?

In any case, should the results of this study really be surprising? If we are working in the garden, using long-handled rakes, shovels, and hoes without wearing gloves, the constant rubbing of the rake handle against the skin of our palms will cause that skin to react to protect itself. It will spin out extra skin cells, which will dry out and become a protective callus that will persist as long as the irritating force (the rake handle) continues to rub against the skin. If gloves are worn, or garden work is finished and the skin on the palm is no longer rubbed by the rake handle, the callus skin will soften and recede.

We know that cigarette smokers, whose lung linings are subjected to the same repeated carcinogen exposure as that of our poor medical school rabbit's ears, and whose bronchial mucosa show the same tissue changes steadily progressing to a cancer, are capable of beginning to reverse those changes within weeks of stopping smoking. The South African study showed, in visual detail, that the colon lining can muster the same disease-reversal process, given the low-meat, high-fiber food stream described above. The sooner our GI colleagues stop fearing the cultural taboos about assessing their patient's diet as a causative factor in their disease, the sooner their patients will progress towards true cure of their disease.

Prevention and Reversal of Fatty Liver Disease

Nestled beneath your right lower rib cage is a true wonder of the universe. It is a stunningly complex, brilliantly organized, three-pound mass of purplish tissue known as your liver, and its myriad functions and underlying chemical machinery will take hepatologists decades more to thoroughly grasp, to the extent that such an outcome is even possible. I have boundless respect for the capacity of the human mind, especially when teamed with the rigors of applied science, but I'm not sure that it can ever fully unlock the intricacies of the liver.

Every liver cell is filled with hundreds of enzymes and organelles that transform one organic compound into another in microseconds, a feat the alchemists of old could only imagine with envy. With reproducible alacrity, the protein enzyme aminotransferase, for example, can clip off a three-atom ammonia group from an amino acid molecule like alanine, thereby converting it into a keto acid called *pyruvate*, ready to be burned in the mitochondria for energy. The liver truly is the master alchemist of our body, tirelessly transmuting the raw components of our food intake into the precious substrates of life.

Distressingly, this marvelous organ finds itself under relentless attack in America today. Nonalcoholic fatty liver disease (NAFLD), a condition characterized by a buildup of too much fat in the liver, is on the rise, along with a more severe form of the disease called *nonalcoholic steatohepatitis* (NASH), which may lead to swelling and scarring (cirrhosis) of the liver.

When I entered medical school, such insults to the liver were almost always the result of excessive alcohol consumption. In fact, the term "non-alcoholic fatty liver disease" had not yet been coined. But now it is estimated that about 25 percent of Americans have NAFLD.[14] Put another way, about one-quarter of our countrymen have managed to injure their livers significantly through diet to a degree that formerly could be expected to be accomplished only by the excessive consumption of alcohol. One study of over nine thousand asymptomatic adults found at least mild steatosis (the infiltration of liver cells with fat) in more than half of its subjects.[15] As many as one in ten American children may be affected by NAFLD,[16] dramatically increasing their chances of experiencing serious liver disease, such as cirrhosis or liver cancer, and requiring liver transplants during their lifetimes. This is not the kind of change I was hoping to witness during my career in medicine.

What has changed to afflict this precious, vulnerable organ so widely? Before we explain the cause of this modern plague, it helps to understand something about how the liver functions.

Here is a brief survey of what your liver is doing for you, right now, as you read these words.

First, it regulates the level of glucose in our blood, able to raise or lower that level as required. As glucose molecules enter the circulation from our food, the liver can absorb them and assemble them into a storage form, called *glycogen*—an "animal starch," if you will. When needed, the glycogen can be broken up (glycogenolysis) into individual glucose molecules again and put back into the blood. This is essential, since our red blood cells (RBCs) that transport oxygen to our cells require a low but steady level of glucose in the blood for them to stay alive. Prolonged bouts of low blood glucose levels, below 55 mg/dL, will severely damage the RBCs and must be avoided at all costs. It is the liver's job to keep the blood sugar above that level, so it constantly releases a trickle of glucose from its stores of glycogen into the bloodstream to protect the RBCs. Thus the liver has the power to both raise and lower glucose levels as needed.

So how does the liver know what to do when? Hormones released from the walls of the GI tract, the pancreas, and the brain, along with nerve impulses transmitted via the vagus nerve, give the liver its chemical cues to either break down or reassemble glycogen molecules in order to keep the blood sugar levels optimal, thus ensuring that each cell receives its due share of energy.

Beyond its role as the body's glucose guardian, the liver functions as a critical detoxifier, constantly filtering the blood of naturally occurring toxins from food, as well as from drugs and alcohol, rendering them harmless while preparing them for safe elimination, usually by excreting the substances into the bile, where they mix with the food stream and eventually ride out of the body with the feces.

The liver serves also as the body's chief chemist, synthesizing a bountiful array of essential proteins, such as fibrinogen and prothrombin, that are crucial for blood clotting. It synthesizes proteins such as complement proteins and C-reactive protein (CRP), all essential for immune system function. Of supreme importance, the liver synthesizes the most abundant protein in the blood's plasma, albumin, whose essential functions include providing the osmotic pull within the bloodstream to prevent water from leaking out into the tissues (edema). Albumin also buffers metabolic acids, transports hormones and drugs, and neutralizes destructive free radicals. Without all these essential proteins, we might bleed to death from simple lacerations, perish from sepsis from an infected sliver, or drown in pulmonary edema as our blood's water component seeps into our lung tissues.

The liver also plays a pivotal role in fat metabolism by producing bile, a greenish-golden fluid essential for the digestion and absorption of fats. Bile is made by liver cells, then collected and transported through the liver's extensive internal duct system until it is ultimately stored and concentrated in the muscular sac on the underside of the liver: the gallbladder.

When a fatty meal leaves the stomach and enters the duodenum, the first section of the small intestine, the wall of that organ releases a hormone called *cholecystokinin*, which prompts the muscular layer of the gallbladder to contract. This squeezes two to four tablespoons of bile through the common bile duct down into the small intestine, where it mixes with the food. There, the bile attaches to large droplets of fats, mostly triglycerides, which are too big to be absorbed into the bloodstream. Like the detergent it is, bile disperses the fatty globules into much smaller droplets (emulsifying them). This allows the lipase enzymes, released from the pancreas and intestinal wall, to more easily break up the triglyceride molecules into free fatty acids, forms that can be absorbed into the bloodstream and transported to the cells that need them.

The liver also regulates the blood level of a pigment called *bilirubin*, a byproduct of the breakdown of old red blood cells. Bilirubin gives bile its characteristic gold-green color and, as it is excreted down the common bile duct and mixed with the food mass, it gives feces its brown color, as well as its feculent aroma.

When the liver cells are sick, as in viral or alcoholic hepatitis, or when the bile duct is obstructed by a gallstone or tumor, the bilirubin is not removed from the bloodstream. The bile backs up into the blood and deposits into the skin and the whites of the eyes (the sclera), where the yellow glow of jaundice signals a problem.

As if these "normal" functions were not impressive enough, the liver's ability to regenerate itself—to regrow from a remnant as small as a quarter of its original size—is nothing short of miraculous. In the operating room, I once witnessed a liver that had about three-quarters of its mass blown away by a shotgun blast; I wondered if the owner of that liver could survive. Ten months later, he returned to the hospital with an intra-abdominal infection requiring us to open him up again. My colleagues and I were stunned to see that his liver had almost completely regenerated in size and shape, as good as new.

Even the liver's blood supply bespeaks the efficiency and ingenuity of the body. A main function of the liver is to assemble the building blocks of protein—the amino acids in our food—into our essential proteins like albumin and fibrinogen. As the digestive enzymes from our pancreas and intestinal wall liberate the amino acids in our food, the amino acids are absorbed by the tiny intestinal villi, microscopic fingerlike projections that protrude into the intestinal channel (the lumen).

The millions of villic veins join with each other to form a spider-web-like network of veins within the intestinal wall that absorb nutrients all along the twenty-two-foot length of the small intestine. These veins continue to join each other until they form the portal vein. "Portal" means "doorway" and, indeed, the portal vein enters the liver through a crease on the undersurface of the organ, called the *porta hepatis*, the doorway into the liver.

Once in the liver, the veins subdivide once more into a vast network of intrahepatic vessels that bathe the liver cells in the nutrient-rich blood, bringing them all the nutrients necessary to accomplish their vital metabolic missions of synthesizing, excreting, and detoxifying the blood.

It is important to keep in mind that, thanks to this ingenious plumbing arrangement, within minutes of eating anything, molecules of that food bathe all of our liver cells. This includes molecules of ethyl alcohol, the active ingredient in beer, wine, and hard liquor. Alcohol, as a chemical, is notorious for killing any cell with which it comes into contact. So within a few minutes of drinking alcohol in any form, it is bathing every precious liver cell, exerting its toxic effects.

The liver cells have enzymes, such as alcohol dehydrogenase, that can detoxify limited amounts of ethyl alcohol. But if the toxic booze baths continue frequently, mechanisms to excrete fats from the liver cells are inhibited, so fats begin to accumulate within the liver cells. This causes the characteristic fatty degeneration of the liver ("fatty liver") that can be seen on ultrasound and MRI scans—and certainly under the pathologist's microscope.

With continued drinking, this condition can progress to permanent scarring and, eventually, internal contracture of the liver known as *cirrhosis*. With bile ducts and blood vessels within the liver permanently distorted, kinked, and obstructed by scar tissue, fatal liver failure is often the result. Fortunately, the liver is the body's champion organ when it comes to healing itself if given the chance. As soon as the repeated toxic tides of alcohol cease, the liver cells repair the damage and the fatty appearance vanishes. Fatty liver is, indeed, reversible, and this should come as a great relief—and treatment guide—also for those afflicted with nonalcoholic fatty liver disease from its fasting-growing cause: diet.

In this now common malady, the culprit is not repeated floods of ethyl alcohol but, rather, recurring surges of refined fructose. Here I must state that I am in complete agreement with Dr. Robert Lufkin, whose book, *Lies I Taught in Medical School*,[17] contains a riveting chapter on the history of fatty liver disease and particularly the sudden emergence of the scourge of NAFLD beginning in the 1980s. Dr. Lufkin condemns the ingestion of fructose in any other form besides that found in whole fruits and vegetables, and his warnings against eating processed, isolated fructose—especially in commercial soft drinks, baked goods, and candies—are well-founded. There are at least three reasons not to consume fructose-loaded treats:

1. Such food-like substances flood prodigious amounts of fructose through every tissue in the body, where it sticks to ("glycosylates") vital protein molecules, like structural collagen and oxygen-carrying hemoglobin, making them stiff, thus prone to fracture and loss of function.
2. The glycosylated proteins can also be oxidized into advanced glycation end products (AGEs) that teem with free radicals, ripping electrons off nearby atoms, wreaking molecular damage on vital structures, and driving aging in all tissues.
3. The liver is essentially the only organ that can metabolize fructose (our muscles don't have the enzymes to burn it for energy) and, even in its healthiest state, the liver has but a limited ability to metabolize much fructose. As the fructose floods overwhelm the hepatic enzymes that can metabolize the sugar, the liver

> tissue is forced to turn the fructose into triglycerides that then accumulate in the cells, spawning the increasing medical scourge of nonalcoholic fatty liver disease, now the most common cause of liver failure in nondrinkers today.

Since every molecule of table sugar is 50 percent fructose, I would urge people to satisfy their sweet tooth with natural treats like mango chunks and grapes, rather than commercial sodas and ultra-processed, sugar-riddled junk foods. We know that the modest amounts of fructose in whole plant foods, which come packaged with a bounty of vitamins, minerals, and water to aid in their metabolism, impose essentially no metabolic burden upon the liver or other organs; they should be daily features of your diet. These same fruits and vegetables also provide fiber that slows down the absorption of fructose and promotes its elimination in the stool.

Fortunately, even when the liver cells in NAFLD have become choked with triglycerides that inhibit vital enzyme functions, all that is required is for the owner of the liver to adopt the diet they should have been eating all along: one based on naturally low-fat, whole plant foods. On this leaner, cleaner fuel mixture, the inflammatory state subsides, and fats that have already been larded into the liver cells are burned for energy. As the weeks go by, meal after whole plant meal, the phytonutrients in vegetable-rich soups, colorful salads, hearty stews, and steamed greens help clear the stored lipids out of the hepatocytes, and the liver returns to its previous, healthy state. Now the liver can again carry out its functions of regulating glucose levels in the bloodstream, excreting waste, and synthesizing essential proteins.

While fructose may well be, as Dr. Lufkin theorizes, the leading cause of the current scourge of NAFLD, the last thing that a person with a fatty liver needs is a fatty Western diet, such as the keto diet that Dr. Lufkin endorses, to add more fat to a liver that needs to clear itself of fat. Instead, a low-fat WPF diet should be the recommended therapy.

Prevention and Partial Reversal of Alzheimer's Disease

A growing body of evidence exists that leads one to conclude that Alzheimer's disease (AD) should be considered a foodborne disease. Although the disease is not wholly attributable to atherosclerotic plaque formation, the cerebral arteries and the blood vessels of AD patients' brains are generally not normal, with thickened walls and signs of free-radical damage. The arteries of AD patients also appear to have many of the same traits as standard atherosclerotic cerebrovascular disease seen in "vascular dementia," which is dementia brought on by restricted blood flow to the brain.

Over 133,000 people were observed in a study examining the relationship between red meat consumption and cognitive health. The 2025 study, published in *Neurology*, found that a mere quarter serving or more of processed red meats—that's about an ounce of corned beef, say—per day was associated with a 13 percent increased risk of dementia.[18] Keep in mind that most people who eat processed meats eat more than a quarter serving.

A bombshell study by Dr. Dean Ornish published in 2024 in the journal *Alzheimer's Research and Therapy* has, with good reason, generated an extraordinary amount of media buzz and interest.[19] This simple but impressive pilot study, conducted on fifty-one patients, may give hope to millions. (Please note that it is only with early-stage dementia that improvements have been documented; no one is claiming to reverse full-blown dementia.)

Those fifty-one patients, all between the ages of forty-five and ninety, and all of whom had been diagnosed with mild cognitive impairment or early dementia, were randomly assigned to either an intervention group (twenty-six patients) or to a control group (twenty-five patients). The intervention group was placed on what was essentially a WPF diet (although that term was not used), supplemented with omega-3 fatty acids with curcumin, multivitamins, coenzyme Q10, vitamin C, vitamin B-12, magnesium, a mushroom powder, and probiotics.

Four standard measures of cognition and function (Clinical Global Impression of Change, Alzheimer's Disease Assessment Scale, Clinical Dementia Rating–Sum of Boxes, and Clinical Dementia Rating Global) were used to evaluate the two cohorts over twenty weeks. In all four measures, the intervention group significantly outperformed the control group. Further, the microbiomes of the intervention group improved, with population increases in the taxa (groups of microorganisms) that are associated with reduced dementia risk and population decreases in those associated with increased dementia risk. Various other biomarkers also showed significant improvements in the intervention group.

The surprise to me is that any of this should be surprising. All the same, Dr. Sanjay Gupta should be congratulated for his effective efforts in the media to bring attention to Dr. Ornish's study, as it offers so much hope for reversing cognitive decline. "What is good for the heart is almost certainly good for the brain," Dr. Gupta said.[20]

Of course it is. Arteries run to both organs, and the food stream's biochemical bullies that threaten the body's arteries do not selectively and benevolently isolate any of our most vital arteries to shield from their mayhem.

A 2023 study published in the *American Journal of Alzheimer's Disease & Other Dementias* was essentially a dissection of multiple waves of data from the National Health and Aging Trends Study (NHATS), conducted by the Johns Hopkins Bloomberg School of Public Health, which gathers information on Medicare recipients via in-person interviews.[21] Teasing out data from NHATS on body mass index, obesity, and cognitive decline, the study "analyzed the impact of obesity on conversion from cognitively normal to MCI [mild cognitive impairment], then dementia, and eventually, death."

The study concluded that:

> [D]ementia is linked to several markers of microvascular endothelial dysfunction. First, dementia is more common in those with congestive heart failure, and cerebral ischemia and stroke cause hypoxia, amyloid-beta deposition [plaques in the brain], and BBB [blood-brain barrier] dysfunction, leading to neurodegeneration. Second, CVD may cause amyloid-beta deposition and influence the age at which ADRD [Alzheimer's disease and related dementias] develops, whereas amyloid-beta can cause cardiovascular deterioration. Third, increased amyloid-beta deposition has also been linked to small infarcts and microbleeds, which often go undiagnosed, thus providing methodological challenges. Fourth, blood vessels in ADRD patients show degenerative alterations, amyloid-beta deposition, and loss of smooth muscle cells. Last, blood vessels with collapsed and deteriorated endothelia are seen in more than 90% of ADRD patients and co-occur with amyloid-beta deposition.

These are simply some of the proposed mechanisms by which cardiovascular disease and Alzheimer's disease are intricately intertwined. Endothelial dysfunction lies at the root of both.

Multiple studies have associated higher saturated fat intake with cognitive decline.[22]

That is why, in Dr. Ornish's words, "The same lifestyle changes [that] could reverse high blood pressure, high cholesterol, type two diabetes, obesity, early-stage prostate cancer . . . may reverse the progression of early-stage Alzheimer's."[23]

In October 2024, the American Heart Association issued a "scientific statement" on "Cardiac Contributions to Brain Health," in which it made the point that "Cardiovascular diseases are the leading cause of death and disability in the United States and around the world. Emerging evidence shows that the heart and the brain, once considered unrelated organ systems, are interdependent and linked through shared risk factors."[24] The lead author of that scientific statement, Dr. Fernando Testai, professor of neurology and rehabilitation at my alma mater, the University of Illinois College of Medicine in Chicago, elaborated on the AHA's scientific statement to CNN: "Emerging evidence suggests that the bidirectional relationship between the heart and the brain is deeper than we thought. Vascular risk factors associated with cardiac diseases . . . can increase the levels of beta-amyloid in the brain, which is recognized as a key marker of Alzheimer's disease. In return, beta-amyloid has been found in the heart and is associated with cardiac dysfunction."[25]

At what point, I wonder, will the medical establishment acknowledge a pattern, endorse the whole plant food diet that leads to welcome outcomes for both the heart and the brain, and train young doctors to actively encourage it in their patients? How many studies do we need to prove the obvious?

Some twenty years ago, an ex–cattle rancher turned vegan activist, Howard Lyman, wrote these words about the disease he christened "Alzheifer's Disease":

> Like heart disease, dementia has acquired a patina of normalcy only because of many of those around us succumb to it. But I believe that, like heart disease, it is a distinctly abnormal condition brought about by an abnormal diet. In the coming decades, science will probably be able to ascribe a cause to Alzheimer's with the same certainty that it can now ascribe a cause to heart disease. And I firmly believe that it will be the exact same cause: meat.[26]

Overcoming Covid-19

We have examined the mechanisms by which metabolic disorders and cognitive disorders respond to the optimal medical therapy, which is dietary therapy. Surely, though, you might assume, a contagious viral disease like Covid-19 has precious little to do with diet. One contracts the disease, after all, by inhaling (after infected individuals exhale, cough, sneeze, or speak) the aerosol droplets that contain the virus. Vegans are clearly no less prone to inhaling droplets than meat eaters. Finally, you might conclude, we have identified a disease for which dietary intake is irrelevant.

You would be wrong.

It's true that there's no reason to believe that an optimal diet will help prevent you from contracting the disease. But there's every reason to believe that your diet will determine the disease's course in your body. If infected, will you have an experience that could be compared to a mild flu or cold, or will you wind up in a hospital on a respirator, or even dead? That difference in outcomes can be traced to diet.

A study published in the prestigious medical journal *BMJ Nutrition, Prevention & Health* of 568 Covid-19 cases in the United States and five European countries found that those on a plant-based diet had 73 percent lower odds of developing moderate to severe Covid-19.[27] (It found no association between diet and infection, however.) Now imagine a pill or a vaccine that could demonstrate 73 percent lower odds of moderate to severe Covid-19. Imagine if the only "side effects" of that pill or vaccine were reduced cholesterol, reduced blood pressure, reduced inflammation, and healthy weight loss. Surely the Nobel Prize in Medicine would be won by the developer of that pill or vaccine. Surely the chief medical advisor to the president of the United States, as well as the surgeon general of the United States, and the director of the US Centers for Disease Control and Prevention (CDC), would celebrate that development in press conferences, interviews, and any media opportunities they could contrive . . . while doing everything within their power to make that pill or vaccine available to all Americans and to tout its use. But did we see Dr. Anthony Fauci, Dr. Vivek H. Murthy, or Dr. Rochelle Walensky, who held those positions, respectively, during the pandemic, once come forth and tout the plant-based diet as a strategy to reduce Covid-19 risk? We did not. (I'll note that Dr. Murthy has made some comments to the press that indicate that he favors a plant-based diet. But he never spoke out clearly for that diet as a strategy to save one's life during the era of Covid-19—an era that, arguably, we are still in, although the pandemic has dramatically receded.) This was a shameful dereliction of duty on all their parts.

It is likely, of course, that they would have feared losing their jobs if they had spoken up forcefully in this way to help save people's lives.

I'll note that the *BMJ* study was merely reporting the dramatically improved Covid-19 experience of people on a "*plant-based diet*," a term that the study defined to include vegetarian diets (including dairy and eggs) and pescatarian diets (including fish). And still the results were impressive. One could only imagine how much more remarkable the results would be if the study reported results of those on a WPF diet.

Dr. Kim Williams is a cardiologist, past president of the American College of Cardiology, and a friend of mine. When interviewed on various podcasts, he noted that he has never come across a case of a person who ate a WPF diet and died of Covid-19. He said he had asked around to medical colleagues and has yet to uncover such a case. While it's hard to prove a negative, it's my belief, and Dr. Williams's belief as well, that there is no such case. In other words, of the more than 1.2 million deaths attributed to Covid-19 in the United States, it's quite possible that not a single victim was a consistent practitioner of the whole plant food diet. If those who eat a WPF diet are even one-half of one percent of Americans, you would expect some six thousand deaths among our cohort, if diet offered no protection. I can't prove this assertion, but I'll stick my neck out and say that I believe that in fact there were none.

Covid-19 effectively targets the obese, the diabetic, and those with significant inflammation in their bodies. A study of over 43,000 patients under age eighteen with Covid-19 found that children with obesity fell into the highest risk group for hospitalization.[28] Another study concluded that "it has been clearly illustrated that obese patients are potentially more vulnerable to COVID-19 and more contagious than lean patients. The co-morbidities associated with obesity were found to be correlated with a severe clinical course of COVID-19 and increased mortality and high

BMI has been shown to be correlated with hospitalization, the need for mechanical ventilation and non-survival."[29] Not only did the study identify obesity as a risk factor for hospitalization and mechanical ventilation, but it also concluded that "Obese populations have a decreased response to vaccinations" and that "Obesity is associated with a variety of co-morbid conditions that have been shown to be associated with increased morbidity and mortality from COVID-19."[30] It also noted something that doctors know all too well: Obese hospital patients are more difficult to transport, to intubate, and to diagnose.

Layers of fat surrounding the ribs and diaphragm, and within the abdomen, make breathing more difficult. You do not want to be living in a default state of suboptimal breathing capacity when you get hit with an airborne virus like Covid-19 that can cause respiratory distress.

Not only do the obese put their own lives at risk to Covid-19, they also spread the disease more efficiently than those of normal weight. As one international study found, "obesity may be responsible for a higher volume and extended duration of viral shedding."[31]

I love my obese patients, and I vehemently reject the accusation that I am "fat shaming" when I discuss the subject of obesity in a medical context. I fully understand that there can be strong psychological underpinnings and overlays as to why people become and remain obese. It is painfully obvious that we live in an obesogenic society. The food industry has been assiduously producing and promoting the foods filled with fats and sugars that foster obesity—and that is not the fault of the consumer. However, it would not be intellectually honest for me to say anything other than that, from the strictly physiologic point of view, obesity, characterized by pounds of visceral fat in the abdomen pumping out inflammatory cytokines, is a disease state, plain and simple. Nothing good comes of it, and it is a disservice to the 42 percent of our compatriots who suffer from the condition to pretend otherwise—just as it is a disservice to them for their trusted doctors not to advise them to adhere to a WPF diet that could free them of that disease state.

I'm well aware that universal adoption of the WPF diet is something of a pipe dream; let us at the same time recognize that if we could achieve the extraordinary pipe dream of human beings enjoying a diet of plants that is the natural human diet—a diet that I and so many of my friends enjoy immensely and find far superior in countless ways to our previous omnivorous diets—we would see a reduction in obesity of *very nearly 100 percent*.

Yes, with the diet I propose, consisting almost entirely of fiber-rich foods that are not calorically dense, we could make obesity vanish from the American landscape (without the aid of Ozempic and the other GLP-1 agonists, which leave the patient tethered to these expensive drugs indefinitely) while enjoying delicious meals of whole plant foods—in other words, human food. At the same time, the incidence of cardiovascular disease and type 2 diabetes would be reduced well over 90 percent, healthcare costs would plummet, and longevity would increase dramatically.

For some reason, this is apparently too much to hope for.

Possible Prevention of ALS (Lou Gehrig's Disease)

We have seen how metabolic disorders are almost always engendered by dietary choices. We have seen that the etiology of an infectious respiratory disease that brought on a pandemic has nothing to do with diet, but that the course and severity of the disease have everything to do with it. And now we come to an example of a cruel, terminal disease that is not as rare as we would hope: amyotrophic lateral sclerosis (ALS), or Lou Gehrig's disease. It afflicts about one in four hundred individuals.[32] Always fatal, ALS is a neurodegenerative disease that attacks motor neurons and robs the patient of control over their muscles—including, ultimately, the ability to breathe or swallow. In about 90 percent of cases, there is no family history of the disease—therefore, no known or suspected genetic cause.

The etiology of ALS may still be justifiably considered unknown, but we shouldn't be oblivious to the good deal that we *do* know—and the likely implications of that knowledge.

The detective mystery begins in Guam, where, around the 1950s and 1960s, the incidence of the disease was about a hundred times as high as in the rest of the world.[33] While disease clustering like this represents a tragedy for the population involved, scientists are trained to see a silver lining: Such anomalies may help advance our understanding of the disease. Why would the people of Guam be so prone to this awful condition?

Attention was drawn to the cycad trees of Guam, since flour made from the dietary seeds was a staple of the local diet, and since livestock reportedly demonstrated neurological disease after eating the seeds.[34] A neurotoxic nonprotein amino acid called BMAA (beta-N-methylamino-L-alanine) was identified in the seeds. While that discovery might have seemed at first to confirm the theory that the seeds were the culprit, the amount of BMAA in the seeds was found to be so slight that the population would have had to have eaten an ungodly quantity of seeds to ingest enough BMAA to suffer any effect. It turned out that there was another part of the Guamanian diet that was more relevant: fruit bats, also known as flying foxes. The fruit bats ate the same cycad seeds, and the BMAA biomagnified in their tissues.[35,36,37] Then, when the Guamanians ate the fruit bats, they indeed absorbed enough of the dosage of the neurotoxin to develop disease. Guamanians also ate other animals, such as pigs, that fed on the seeds. BMAA was found inside the brain tissues of six native Chamorro people in Guam who died of ALS, as well as in brain specimens of others who died of Alzheimer's.[38]

Here's where the story takes a twist. BMAA was also found inside the brains of Canadians who died of Alzheimer's. Surely, most Canadians had never consumed a fruit bat or even a cycad seed. It was then discovered that the cycad trees don't produce BMAA on their own; rather, it is produced by cyanobacteria (also known as blue-green algae) not only in freshwater and marine habitats but also terrestrial habitats, including the roots of cycad trees, where it is absorbed into their seeds. It turns out that all forms of blue-green algae all over the world produce the neurotoxin; therefore, it is absorbed by fish and shellfish everywhere.

A Vermont public television show called *Made Here* broadcast a powerful, short documentary, *Lake Effect,* concerning clusters of ALS diagnoses around lakes in Vermont and New Hampshire. Around Enfield, New Hampshire, for example, a town with a lake prone to cyanobacteria algal blooms, the incidence of ALS is ten to twenty-five times the expected rate.[39] As the documentary points out, lakes suffer blooms of blue-green algae because of phosphorus loading of waterways. The phosphorus loading can be attributed to manure from animal agriculture, as well as from fertilizer, often used to grow crops to feed to farmed animals. The cyanobacteria then get into the fish, crustaceans, and mollusks, and people who eat those sea creatures are consuming the bio-accumulated neurotoxins.

Every link in the chain that may well result in the genesis of ALS traces back to animal agriculture and the human folly of putting our environment at risk to satisfy our taste for flesh. First, the manure and fertilizer attendant to animal agriculture pollute our waterways and lead to toxic blue-green algae blooms, then we make the mistake of eating the fish, crustaceans, and mollusks that have been contaminated with the toxin.

The problem of blue-green algae blooms is practically ubiquitous and may be at least partially responsible not only for an untold number of cases of ALS but for the global spread of Parkinson's and Alzheimer's as well. As sewage and runoff from animal agriculture pollute waterways, toxic algal blooms are appearing worldwide. A study of biomagnification of BMAA concentrations in aquatic food chains found that "Pink shrimp in Florida Bay . . . have high concentrations of BMAA, comparable to those found in the fruit bats of Guam . . . Pink shrimp and blue crabs in south Biscayne Bay have a wide range of concentrations . . . All three species of fish from the Caloosahatchee River . . . have high concentrations of BMAA similar to that of the fruit bats of Guam."[40] A 1990 study of a cluster of ALS cases in a small town in Wisconsin suggested a link to consumption of Lake

Michigan fish.[41] In 2018, a study was published using meticulous satellite mapping of blue-green algae concentrations in New England to assess relationships with ALS cases. It concluded that "The outcomes support the hypothesis that cyanotoxins increase the risk of ALS, which helps our understanding of the etiology of ALS."[42] In Southern France, in a region known for shellfish production and consumption, a cluster of ALS cases came to light, and high concentrations of BMAA were found in oysters and mussels in the cluster area.[43] It was a similar story with consumption of blue crabs in an area with an ALS cluster by the Chesapeake Bay.[44]

So, you may ask: Has it been established definitively by science that consumption of fish, crustaceans, and mollusks presents a risk of developing ALS—as well as perhaps Alzheimer's and Parkinson's disease?

Well, let me make an analogy here to murder investigations. Sometimes, you hear on the news of a gruesome murder, and you learn that on the day of the killing, police discovered an abandoned van a hundred yards from the body, and they traced its ownership to an individual who had recently escaped from prison and was wanted for murder in a neighboring state. How do the police refer to him? As a "person of interest." Under their professional protocols, the police may feel that it's too soon to call him a "suspect." And of course it's far too soon, under our system of justice, to call him the "killer."

All the same, when I hear facts like those reported on the news, I suspect that when they arrest and prosecute the guy, he's going to turn out to be the killer, and he will be justly convicted. There's not usually an innocent explanation for an escaped convict to abandon a van near a victim's body.

And so a few facts can be true at the same time. First, as I acknowledge, the etiology of ALS (and other neurodegenerative diseases) has not yet been definitively established by science. Second, there could be more than one causal agent at play. It has even been suggested that other toxins in seafood, such as methylmercury, could have a synergistic effect with BMAA.[45] Third, most crucially, *there is extremely good reason, based on the existing evidence, to avoid consumption of all sea creatures in the interest of preventing neurodegenerative disease.*

People need to know this information, so that they can make an informed decision regarding what foods to ingest. Caring doctors should share this information with their patients.

Avoiding Alpha-Gal Syndrome

For decades now, I have lent my voice to a growing chorus of medical doctors and researchers who have encouraged people to shun animal foods and sustain themselves on a nourishing diet of whole plant foods.

It never occurred to me that we might be bolstered in that cause by a tick.

We can't always choose our allies, after all. The lone star tick (*Amblyomma americanum*) inhabits wooded areas in the Midwest and East, and it's so named because of a white, star-shaped spot on the shield of the adult female.

You don't want to get bitten by a lone star tick if you can help it; while it is unlikely to cause Lyme disease, it can transmit other illnesses. Most notably, it can bring on alpha-gal syndrome.

Individuals bitten by the lone star tick produce antibodies to respond to alpha-gal, a sugar molecule foreign to humans but found in non-primate mammalian meat (beef, pork, lamb, venison). These antibodies may bring on, a few hours after eating red meat, an allergic reaction that sickens those tick-bitten meat eaters. The reaction can take the form of itching, swelling, nausea, vomiting, diarrhea, or even severe anaphylaxis.

While I appreciate that the lone star tick may be trying only to improve our health and encourage us to treat our fellow creatures with more compassion, prevent pandemics, and save the planet, this is not the method that I would choose to steer people away from meat.

Still, those following a plant-based diet have far less to worry about, should they cross paths with this unexpected emissary of dietary change.

Chapter Five

THE REASONS THE ESTABLISHMENT RESISTS

"Why doesn't my doctor know anything about nutrition?"

I seem to encounter this question several times each month. In patient consultations and in their medical emails to me, in media articles and in interviews with other physicians, in my conversations with medical colleagues, and when reading articles published in medical journals, the lack of nutritional training and understanding among doctors and our allied health professionals reveals itself to be stunningly, embarrassingly evident. Medical schools, medical boards, and practicing physicians all seem to willfully disregard the potent role that whole plant foods can play in reversing chronic disease. But why is this so?

The resistance from each of these powerful entities to opening the intellectual doors even a crack to the healing power of foods is manifold—and seemingly adamantine. From universities, to hospitals, to clinicians' offices, to mega-profitable insurance companies, the status quo holds, firmly cemented in place by a tenacious bond of money, politics, and culture, as the very role of physicians diminishes behind a fortress of bureaucracy and paperwork.

Meanwhile, the health of the American people deteriorates, by all measurable metrics, seemingly by the year, as our girth increases.

Our medical establishment today has no difficulty linking smoking to lung cancer, but it resisted the obvious for a shameful length of time in the 1950s and 1960s; it took some seven thousand scientific articles linking cigarette smoking to lung cancer to convince the medical authorities at the time to certify, and act upon, that causality.[1] As Dr. Michael Greger, founder of NutritionFacts.org, is wont to say, "You'd think six thousand studies might have been enough."

Smoking had been socially acceptable before science spoiled the "fun" of lighting up. On the other hand, abusing alcohol, especially hard liquor, never enjoyed as much social approval as smoking, and that may be why there was never any resistance, as far as I know, to establishing the fact that alcoholics often drink their way into cirrhosis of the liver. Prolific alcohol consumption was always spurned and lamented by society, so the medical truth of its harm to the liver had no trouble emerging.

Eating animal foods is a habit that enjoys far more public support today, and involves an industry that has amassed far more power than smoking or drinking ever enjoyed. The suppression of the painfully obvious fact that human beings eat their way into heart disease, hypertension, type 2 diabetes, autoimmune conditions, some forms of cancer, and many other diseases has continued unabated for decades. It represents, if you will, the pièce de résistance of medical resistance.

Most people in our society, after all, eat animal products. They were fed those foods by loving parents, and they have seen those foods promoted by advertising in every communication and information medium they encounter. Most of the doctors and other health professionals they visit do not object to the consumption of animal foods, or may even, as a consequence of nutritional ignorance, actively promote it. These foods are offered in abundance in restaurants, schools, and even hospitals. Yes, hospitals blithely serve meat to heart attack patients, whose meat eating bought them their ticket to the hospital in the first place. Obscenely, you can even find McDonald's establishments inside some hospitals; there are some eighteen hospitals in America with fast-food franchises conveniently drumming up more hospital business inside their walls.[2]

Millions of our countrymen are employed in jobs that, in one way or another, involve the production and distribution of animal foods. Very nearly half the land mass of the United States is devoted to producing animal foods. In short, nothing could be more normal in America than eating animal foods. The brave minority of medical professionals who attempt to follow the science, which points overwhelmingly to the reality that animal foods do considerable harm to the human body, are forced to navigate a minefield of resistance that dwarfs the onetime formidable resistance to acknowledging the truth of the harms of cigarette smoking.

The healthcare system, in its present form, represents a behemoth of a foe to all who dare imagine that it could actually be transformed into a benevolent agent that helps us in our healing and keeps injury or illness from diminishing our futures.

Culture and Cuisine

The underlying resistance to change stems from our culture itself. Culture shapes us powerfully; it's generally viewed as a wonderful, nurturing, benevolent influence on our lives. We are virtually all proud of our various cultures, whether that culture is African American, Chinese, French, Greek, Hispanic, Irish, Italian, Japanese, Jewish, Native American, Polish, or what have you. Within the United States, there's often regional pride as well: Southern pride, Appalachian pride, New England pride. All of these ethnicities and regions boast unique cuisines.

Not one of which is vegan.

How do you explain to a person of Greek ancestry that the salad they are enjoying would be far healthier without the fatty feta cheese? How do you explain to a person of Japanese ancestry that consuming fish-based sushi presents a risk of neurological disease? How do you explain to a person with German roots that their bratwurst will likely lead to weight gain and a heart attack? Or to a Southerner that their fried comfort foods are slowly killing them? Or to a Jewish person that pastrami is a Group 1 carcinogen? Or to an African American that the chitlins and pigs' feet they may celebrate in their culture were introduced to their diet as the scraps that their enslaved ancestors of not so long ago were disdainfully permitted to eat in the South, while their more distant, free ancestors in Africa ate far better, usually plant-based food?

The American culture, which pushes greasy, salty fast food and sugary desserts while normalizing obesity, washes over all the ethnic cultures that blend into our melting pot, exacerbating all that may already be wrong, from a health perspective, with their traditional cuisines.

How do you make the case that cultures are not perfect and may in some ways be harming their faithful and loving adherents? How do you make the case that the traditional cuisine on which a person was raised since childhood is clogging his arteries or raising her blood pressure?

You can readily see why most physicians consider navigating these cultural minefields beyond their scope of duty.

Keep in mind, too, that practicing physicians and those who run medical schools may well be as attached to their cultural cuisines as anyone else. I understand that. Yes, I was appalled by it on that fateful day during my anesthesiology residency in Vancouver when I watched that obese surgeon wolf down a burger, milkshake, and fries after performing heart surgery—but I was the only one on the surgical team so appalled.

Vegans are outliers, after all, in American culture. Adopting a plant-based diet may feel like abandoning the winning side for the losing side, the popular club for the unpopular club.

I grant all that. Still, there is a professional obligation, when you are a doctor or a medical school director, to *follow the science*, even when it contradicts cherished cultural traditions.

Doctors can start by challenging themselves to change their own diets—much as I did, enthusiastically, when I embraced the hearty plant-based food at the Gentle World community and watched my excess pounds melt away. It was the best decision I ever made.

Let's not forget the guideline that every physician strives to follow: First, do no harm.

Allow me to extend that concept from medical treatments to daily habits. You harm yourself every time you put an animal-based food or fried food or donut into your mouth. If you, as a doctor, make a habit of harming yourself this way, you will lose credibility in counseling your patients on their diets. That will make you more reluctant to even raise the subject of diet—and that reluctance in turn *harms your patient* who may need your nutritional counsel, if you are qualified to give it.

This turns out to be especially true if the physician is overweight or obese. Back in 2007, the Physicians' Health Study of nineteen thousand doctors found that 40 percent were overweight and 23 percent were obese.[3] One effect of overweight and obesity in physicians turns out to be that, according to a 2018 study, "non-obese physicians were more likely to document obesity, and documentation of obesity lagged significantly in comparison to hypertension."[4] The study further concluded that "Prior studies suggest that documentation rates of obesity are low for several reasons, including a physician's own bias to recognize obesity. In addition, as stated previously, although most physicians believe obesity is a disease, they may not document it because they feel efforts at addressing obesity are futile."[5]

Really? It's futile to address a disease state that can lead to death by heart attack, stroke, cancer, and other killers? It's a safe assumption, borne out by this study, that it's more likely to seem futile to address obesity if you, the doctor, are overweight or obese yourself. That is why there is a professional obligation, in my view, to set a good example. That means following the science in your life as well as in your practice—and yes, sorry, but that often means upsetting the apple cart of cultural tradition.

The Hole in Our Knowledge

The first step in the direction of moving medicine forward would be to post some illuminated signs in medical schools that say *Follow the Science.*

If, in the months after I graduated medical school, the present-day me had materialized in a puff of vapor in the office of the newly minted, twenty-four-year-old Dr. Klaper, and began quizzing the young me with nutrition-based questions about protein requirements, fiber requirements, antioxidant sources, folate sources, carotenoid sources, glucosinolates in cruciferous vegetables, anthocyanins in berries, prebiotics and probiotics, the role of fermented foods, or the need for vitamin D3 and vitamin B12 supplementation, most every query would have left my younger self slack-jawed and silent. I had only recently graduated from the University of Illinois College of Medicine in Chicago, long recognized as one of the finest medical schools in the country—yet there I was, a nutritional know-nothing, skilled in writing intravenous orders to keep a person alive with synthetic fluids, but absent a clue as to what to tell a functioning human being to eat in order to stay healthy, let alone to turn around killer diseases like hypertension and type 2 diabetes. How and why was I unleashed upon an unsuspecting public absolutely bereft of knowledge as to how to use the most powerful tool any physician can wield to overcome disease and allay suffering in our patients? Where was the hole in the knowledge net that let this massive asset slip through and sink to the bottom, unseen and unutilized—and how do we fix the hole?

In medical education, it seems the reluctance of North American medical schools to include plant-based nutrition in their curricula is influenced by a variety of systemic, cultural, and practical factors, starting with its historical focus on pharmacology and disease treatment.

The traditional medical education model in North America has long been focused on *treating* diseases rather than *preventing* them. Consequently, most medical schools prioritize pharmacology, surgical interventions, and acute care, leaving scarcely any room for nutrition education.

Medical curricula are heavily grounded in a biomedical approach, which emphasizes the physiological and biochemical mechanisms of disease and often views nutrition as secondary to pharmaceutical solutions. Medical schools nurture the attitude often expressed in the surgical suites: *"Nutrition is a sissy science. We're in this operating room doing real medicine!"*

Those who think that way suffer from a false sense of medical superiority. For in that operating room, they are generally dealing with the infections, infarctions, and amputations that stem from what their patients have been eating. Whether they realize it or not, they are more often than not treating nutrition-based diseases—many, if not most, of which could have been prevented or even reversed with adherence to a whole plant food diet. Sadly, with the "nutrition doesn't make a difference" mindset, the notion of plant-based nutrition at best aligns more with preventive medicine, which is readily dismissed as having no legitimate place in an active medical clinic. The reversibility of disease through nutrition is not considered an option; it was, after all, never taught to doctors.

As a result of their medical education, too many doctors—and, most urgently, too many *family doctors*—view their primary function to be addressing illnesses in their patients rather than informing them as to how to stay healthy.

Not a Conspiracy, But . . .

Now we come to the tricky and nuanced subject of money, and how its incentives play out in the medical system.

Let me be clear that I don't believe that most of my colleagues are shallow, greedy, malevolent hucksters and swindlers looking to maximize their own profit and earnings at the expense of their patients. Most physicians are honorable people. I don't believe that the problem with most cardiologists, for example, is that they say to themselves, "Gee, I could easily help save my patient's life by explaining and encouraging the whole plant food diet, but there's more money to be made with surgical interventions, so let's start with an angioplasty and then hopefully move on up to a heart bypass, all of which will reward my pocketbook handsomely, the patient's health and life be damned."

That's not the case. Gastroenterologists do not recommend colonoscopies that they believe are not in their patients' best interest, and radiologists don't order imaging just for the hell of it, in order to make money.

In short, I don't believe that there's a conscious conspiracy of greed between medical schools, physicians, medical device manufacturers, hospitals, clinics, and insurance companies to maximize profits at the expense of their patients.

But I *do* believe that there are financial incentives that play out in such a way that—even with each physician and each participant in an intertwined, complex medical system doing what they may believe, in good conscience, to be in the best interest of patients—costs tend to be maximized, the payer (patient, insurance company, government/taxpayer, or some combination of the above) tends to pay more than should be necessary, doctors tend to be remunerated at least satisfactorily (and sometimes quite handsomely), and health outcomes are suboptimal. What we are left with is not a conspiracy of greed, but an inefficient and ineffective system that, to a cynical eye, acutely resembles one.

How does this happen?

We start, again, with medical schools. As explained above, these hallowed institutions disregard nutrition as irrelevant to their mission of educating future doctors. It doesn't help that many medical schools receive significant funding from pharmaceutical companies and food industry stakeholders; these same entities also help to fund medical journals, medical conferences, continuing medical education programs, and medical research. Within medical schools, these "charitable" actors can subtly or directly influence the curriculum content that is taught to the students. They needn't make much of an effort, though, as they generally have no reason to be discontent with the status quo. I'm guessing that they know very well that a shift towards plant-based nutrition would challenge the profitability of animal agriculture, and it would reduce the pharmaceutical interventions required to address diet-related illnesses, but it takes little effort to forestall that shift.

The National Board of Medical Examiners has essentially no nutrition questions on the National Board exams beyond testing the student's awareness of some nutrient deficiency syndromes (which most doctors will never see) and some general nutrition principles—but nothing concerning how to use the patient's diet to prevent or arrest chronic disease. This, then, drives a vicious cycle, permitting the medical schools to say, "Until the National Board starts putting nutrition questions on the Board exams, we're not going to clutter up our curriculum with nutrition courses." The patient's diet as a cause and potential cure of disease thereby remains unmentioned and invisible. It seems that both the National Board of Medical Examiners and the medical schools think that no one is watching and that no one cares. The public, however, as we shall see, is starting to care.

Doctors embarking on their careers understandably deduce that nutrition couldn't possibly have a great deal of relevance to health, or else someone might have bothered to mention the subject in medical school. As those careers play out, many soon feel compelled to practice "defensive medicine," ordering tests and procedures of questionable necessity, as they fear that they might get sued if they take no such action and the patient experiences a bad outcome. Ordering those tests and procedures is often considered the "standard of care." They are therefore kept mightily busy doing everything but dealing with the underlying health of their patients.

Most of those patients have been passively trained to expect such medical treatments as drugs or surgeries when they enter the healthcare system. A significant portion of patient satisfaction derives from receiving what they perceive as tangible, immediate treatments, rather than long-term lifestyle recommendations. Patients tend to view medical visits as an opportunity to get some problem "fixed" rather than an opportunity to learn how to regain their health. Encouraging patients to adopt a WPF diet requires ongoing support, education, and follow-up, none of which is accommodated by our fee-for-service medical model. If you run a for-profit institution, perennially focused on patient satisfaction scores and reimbursement models, you likely would view WPF nutrition as a disincentive to your bottom line, and you might have some justification in arguing that you are instead providing the sort of care that patients want.

What about the hospitals? About 25 percent of hospitals are for profit, so they can't be expected to jump upon any health reform bandwagon in an effort to create a healthier population that might leave their premises and surgical suites half empty. Nonprofit hospitals have incentives that are not much different; while their nonprofit status allows them to receive tax-deductible donations, they can be as focused as for-profit hospitals on the bottom line. In theory, nonprofit hospitals may be more likely to be concerned with providing services to the community that may not be particularly profitable, such as psychiatric services, but that's not always the case. Nonprofit hospitals, too, need to bring in revenue from patients, with the subtle distinction that their excess revenue is accounted for as "net income" rather than "profit." The "net income" can be used to hire more staff, raise salaries, or add to the hospital's endowment funds. So for-profit hospitals seek higher profit, while not-for-profits seek higher net income—a distinction that may seem, as far as the public is concerned, more or less theoretical, and not particularly relevant to patient experience.

Hospitals invest heavily in advanced medical technology and procedures (e.g., angioplasty, heart bypass surgery, organ transplants, and bariatric surgeries). These treatments are lucrative, both in terms of billing insurance (and patients) and attracting patients. Often, lifelong post-interventional care is necessary and contributes to an ongoing income stream from such procedures. A WPF diet could prevent the need for many of these interventions, directly threatening these income streams. The strong relationships between hospitals and medical device companies create an additional layer of resistance to any change that might decrease demand for costly procedures and devices.

Even if a maverick hospital, unconcerned with the prospect that nutritional therapy might cost it considerable income from reduced need for cardiac surgery, bariatric surgery, and more, wanted to promote plant-based diets, that would require retraining healthcare staff, something that hospitals are ill-equipped to do. It's far easier to continue to undervalue nutrition and leave preventive dietary interventions sidelined. It's the rare hospital that even cares to make the most obvious and minimal nutritional effort that it could and should make: serving healthy meals to its patients. Most of those rare hospitals are clustered in New York City, where all eleven city-run hospitals have actually saved money by offering a plant-based meal as the primary dinner option, and patient satisfaction has been over 90 percent.[6] But in most hospitals in America, health is not on the menu. Instead, with stunning callousness bordering on outright cruelty, roast beef sandwiches on white bread are served to cardiac patients shortly after their heart attacks.

Medical device makers surely have no financial interest in diminishing need for their products, whether we're talking about blood glucose monitors or stents or robotic surgical systems.

Behind all these institutions stand individual human beings who are no different than anyone else—and no less influenced by their culture. Most stakeholders in this medical establishment grew up in America, a nation that devotes half of its land mass to animal agriculture, while celebrating cowboys, Thanksgiving turkey, ice cream, hamburgers, hot dogs, French fries, and milkshakes. Those raised in foreign cultures likely grew up cherishing animal-based foods as well. Children in America who will one day become doctors and nurses and medical school professors see the same billboards and watch the same advertisements for fast-food chains as children who will one day become ballet dancers; the only difference is that the future ballet dancers have better reason to defy those advertisements and lay off the fast food. You can still succeed handsomely in your career, on the other hand, if you become an obese doctor.

The Truth About Insurance Companies

And then there are the insurance companies, those unloved bureaucratic institutions that, doctors often complain, do all but call the shots in their working lives. I used to naively believe that insurance companies could stun the world by becoming an unlikely force for genuine health reform that could lead to a more fit and vital population. What gave me that outlandish idea?

Health insurance companies, I reasoned, have a clear financial incentive to promote whole-food, plant-predominant nutrition. After all, such an eating style can help prevent and reverse most chronic diseases, thus reducing the healthcare costs that these companies are compelled to cover, at least in part. Surely, they should be interested in paying out fewer claims for hospitalized inpatients and clinic outpatients. It made instinctive sense to think that, if the population got healthier and presented fewer medical insurance claims, the insurance companies would earn greater profits. Their shareholders would be delighted that they could retain more cash at the end of the year. Most of these companies do, after all, pay some lip service to "healthy diet and lifestyle" in their advertising brochures. All they needed to do was to act effectively in support of "healthy diet and lifestyle," rather than merely giving the idea token and vague encouragement. A good start would be making those brochures more informative, by stressing consumption of plant foods over animal foods and whole foods over processed foods. Insurance companies could sponsor classes and lectures on plant-based nutrition; doing so becomes easier and less expensive, in fact, in a world gone virtual. Perhaps they could even financially incentivize participation in plant-based programs, events, and courses. If we could only convince insurance companies that it would be in their own best interest to spread the plant-based gospel . . . well, you can see my naive train of thought.

Alas, that idea proved a bit simplistic. The health insurance industry's profit margin is currently about 3.4 percent.[7] It stays in that range year over year. Under the Affordable Care Act ("Obamacare"), there are medical loss ratio rules: Claim payments must account for at least 80 percent of a health insurance company's revenue for individual and small-group plans, and at least 85 percent for large-group plans. Any profit must come out of the remaining 15 to 20 percent, but of course there's enormous overhead involved in processing claims, marketing insurance plans, and paying insurance agents. Insurance companies are left with that relatively slim profit margin of 3.4 percent.

Of course, 3.4 percent of a giant number can still mean huge profit and rewards for shareholders. Elevance Health (formerly Anthem) grew its revenue from about $59 billion in 2010 to over $170 billion in 2023.[8] Insurance companies can grow their revenue, and therefore their profit, in two ways: by gaining more customers and by raising premiums—but the latter strategy must be justified by higher claims. A sicker population means more claims, justifying higher insurance premiums, leading to higher revenues, and likely the same 3.4 percent profit margin on a higher gross. A healthier population that made fewer claims would inevitably result—given a competitive marketplace and the Obamacare regulations—in health insurance companies being forced to lower their premiums and therefore their revenues and profits.

In short, insurance companies clearly aren't going to lead us out of this mess.

Will the ongoing research into nutrition overwhelm all these forces of resistance so that finally the bold, clear facts supporting plant-based nutrition will speak for themselves and the medical schools will at last bend to follow the science?

Don't hold your breath. Much of the funding for research into nutrition comes, again, from Big Pharma, as well as industries with interests in the consumption of dairy, meat, and processed foods. While the overwhelming majority of nutritional studies support the conclusion that eating plant foods leads to better health outcomes, obfuscation continues.

Perhaps most infamously, the "Red Meat Papers," published in the

Annals of Internal Medicine in 2019, endorsed continued red meat consumption, making headlines that confused many and caused keto dieters everywhere to celebrate. The study was a meta-analysis of existing studies on the health implications of eating meat. The authors reviewed existing nutritional research, gave a "weak" grade to much of it, and concluded that people do not have a "willingness to change unprocessed red or processed meat consumption,"[9] and therefore, there was no good reason why they should. As the authors phrased it, "the desirable effects (a potential lowered risk for cancer and cardiometabolic outcomes) associated with reducing meat consumption probably do not outweigh the undesirable effects (impact on quality of life, burden of modifying cultural and personal meal preparation and eating habits)."[10]

In other words, *we've reviewed the lousy evidence, and yes, you may lower your risk of dying from cancer and heart disease by giving up meat, but it's a pain in the ass, so don't bother.*

A respected scientific journal actually published that "study."

Just as clever defense lawyers can manage to defend a murderer by invoking technicalities and sowing irrational doubts, clever researchers, using little but academic sleight of hand, manage to cobble together and publish studies to defend a meat-based diet that has killed far more people than any murderer ever could.

Studies like the notorious "Red Meat Papers" seem designed to give credence to the fallacy that the science is not yet in on whether animal foods bring on disease and whether plant foods are more salubrious. Studies this dubious are rare, though. More respectable science continues valiantly knocking on the door every day. It's the medical establishment that's responding, "Nobody's home."

The reality is that the healthcare system has long been oriented towards treating illness through reactive measures—pharmaceuticals, surgeries, and other interventions—rather than focusing on prevention. Promoting a WPF diet as a primary tool for disease prevention would require a significant cultural shift within healthcare institutions and educational institutions. Institutional inertia, driven by entrenched practices and habits, along with perverse financial incentives, makes adopting new approaches like plant-predominant (or, better yet, plant-exclusive) nutrition challenging.

Change from the Ground Up

Imagine a dean of a medical school who becomes sympathetic to plant-based nutrition and understands the importance of teaching the subject to the students in her charge. Perhaps her own personal health journey led her to understand the value of plant-based nutrition, and she realizes how important it would be for all doctors to learn about the reversibility of disease through diet therapy. She becomes determined to surmount all the obstacles to teaching nutrition to medical students. Consider the challenges such a WPF-diet-friendly dean would face. She would almost certainly face internal political opposition to any changes she wanted to make to the curriculum. Incorporating a new curriculum requires significant resources for developing, implementing, and evaluating the courses, so funding could be a problem. She would undoubtedly run into the common objection that medical curricula are already densely packed, with limited room for additional courses. (*Where in the schedule are we supposed to put the nutrition course? What course do we drop to make room for it? Surgery? Pathology?*) She might have trouble finding a qualified professor to teach the new courses, although with the explosion in plant-based physicians and dietitians in this country, that challenge could well be met. Still, all in all, it could be a lonely task for such a dean to take on that challenge, and she might well put her position and salary at risk.

For all these reasons, medical schools and the medical establishment at large continue to resist the mountain of science that informs us that a diet of whole plant foods will help both to prevent and to reverse disease.

The revolution, if it is to come, will need to come from the ground up, as young doctors in medical school manage on their own—or with the help of our nonprofit education initiative, Moving Medicine Forward—to learn the truth about the power of plant-based nutrition, and as the general population learns this lesson and brings it to the attention of their doctors. Here are some steps we all can take to bring about much-needed change (and see my "Action Plan for Medical Professionals and Members of the Public," at the end of this book, for more).

To the lay public, I say: Know that your doctor is likely more or less ignorant about how your diet may be harming you and how to help you use diet to create better health. That is a travesty that needs to be addressed. On the positive side, *just by reading this book*, you will likely know far more about nutrition than your doctor, and you will have a good idea about how to use nutrition to prevent and reverse disease.

To young doctors, I ask: Did you spend years in medical school just to become another cog in the medical-industrial machine—a system that hands out pills for lifestyle-induced diseases while staying silent about the root cause?

If you're not talking to your patients about nutrition, exercise, sleep, and real prevention and reversal of disease, you are not practicing medicine—you're just managing decline.

Educate yourself. Please watch my lecture, "What I Wish I Learned About Nutrition in Medical School" (viewable at MovingMedForward.org). Learn about and join the American College of Lifestyle Medicine (lifestylemedicine.org) and the Plantrician Project (plantricianproject.org).

Set a good example for your patients, your colleagues, your family, and your friends. Live your best, healthiest, most joyful life. Eat a whole plant food diet, walk outside every day, get restorative sleep, avoid alcohol and tobacco use, manage your stress, do some meaningful service every day, spend time in nature, and bring as much love into your life as you can.

That will give you a great advantage in helping your patients do the same.

Chapter Six

THE ZEITGEIST

In May 2022, Democratic Congressman Jim McGovern of Massachusetts and Republican Congressman Michael Burgess of Texas (himself formerly a doctor of obstetrics and gynecology) co-sponsored a resolution that called for medical schools to provide nutrition education that would teach medical students the connection between diet and disease. The good news is that the resolution passed the House.[1] The bad news is that, as a mere resolution, it was toothless; it served simply as a statement of sentiment, not as a binding piece of legislation.

You can be certain that its co-sponsors, the liberal congressman from Massachusetts and the conservative now-former congressman from Texas, agree on very little else. But they do agree that, at long last, nutrition should be taught in medical schools.

Everyone wants this madness to end, even members of Congress—Democrats and Republicans.

In the words of Dr. Stephen Devries, a cardiologist who is co-leader of the Harvard T.H. Chan School of Public Health–based Nutrition Education Working Group:

> The burden of diet-related disease is rapidly growing, yet nutrition education of physicians remains sorely lacking. Food is a powerful medicine,

> and like all medicines, physicians need to be proficient in its use. Physicians better trained in nutrition are also much more likely to make referrals to dietitians, a vastly underutilized resource. And for pediatricians, in whose hands we entrust the health and future of our children, the consequences of a lack of sufficient nutrition training are especially alarming. Nutrition is truly the low hanging fruit in medicine . . .[2]

In September 2024, *JAMA Network Open* published a "Consensus Statement" that concerned training physicians in nutrition.[3] A group of thirty-seven experts, including many medical residency directors, was assembled to essentially take a survey about which "nutritional competencies" should be included as part of a medical education and incorporated into licensing and board certification examinations. All thirty-seven agreed, for example, on this proposed competency: "Provides evidence-based, culturally sensitive nutrition and food recommendations to patients for the prevention and treatment of disease." In other words, the experts voted and agreed that doctors should be trained in that competency.

Frankly, I don't know whether to be cheered by this development or to shrug at it. I'm glad that my medical colleagues are discussing the subject of teaching nutrition in medical schools. But the process has a kick-the-can-down-the-road feel to it. What exactly does the "evidence-based, culturally sensitive nutrition" advice that all agree would be worth dispensing look like? Whose ideas about nutrition would be taught? How would the curriculum be designed? When would this ever start?

As of this writing, three of America's premier bestselling works of nonfiction that relate to the way medicine is practiced in this country, all written by practicing physicians, are *Lies I Taught in Medical School*, by Dr. Robert Lufkin; *Good Energy*, by Dr. Casey Means; and *Eat to Beat Disease*, by Dr. William Li. (I'll note that Dr. Lufkin and I share the same publisher, BenBella Books.)

Although we have different medical backgrounds and different beliefs on the subject of nutrition, I agree on a surprising number of health matters with these three gifted authors and dynamic thinkers. Most notably, we all agree that most of the diseases plaguing our population—obesity, heart disease, type 2 diabetes, fatty liver disease, hypertension, and autoimmune conditions—are largely brought on by an unnatural diet, as opposed to genes or bad luck. After reading their books, I feel confident that Drs. Lufkin, Means, and Li would not object to my contention that the tired excuse "Etiology Unknown" should not be applied to any of these conditions. We all believe that these diseases are reversible through diet and lifestyle, and consequently we all believe that to treat these conditions only with pharmaceuticals or surgical interventions, as doctors are trained to do, is to shortchange patients and place their long-term health at risk. We all agree that sugar, refined carbohydrates, seed oils, and processed foods do an enormous amount of harm, and they contribute mightily to obesity and to all these modern plagues. We all see great value in eating whole foods rather than processed foods. We all want consumers to read food labels in a careful and informed way in order to understand what's in their food. We all would like our fellow countrymen to abstain from diet drinks, high-fructose corn syrup, artificial sweeteners, highly processed foods, and junk foods. We are all likewise wary of artificial flavorings, colorings, and preservatives. We all agree that fructose, especially from nonfruit sources, is a hidden danger in our diets. I'll bet that we all agree that vague dietary encouragement, such as to "eat healthy foods," is unhelpful. We all see value in intermittent fasting, and we all believe that *when* you eat is a matter of importance. We all agree that drinking your calories is generally not an optimal dietary strategy. Naturally, we all agree (as do all doctors) on the importance of sleep and exercise and avoidance of harmful substances such as tobacco and alcohol.

And we all share the goal of changing dramatically the way that medicine is practiced in America. We all want to empower individuals to take charge of their own health rather than supinely surrender that responsibility to doctors. Surely, like me, Dr. Means and Dr. Li would enthusiastically sign off on Dr. Lufkin's sage advice that "You can prevent what medicine can only treat."[4] Surely, like me, Dr. Lufkin and Dr. Li would fully endorse Dr. Means's proclamation that "What we put into our bodies is the most critical decision for our health and happiness."[5] I believe we would all affirm Dr. Li's analysis: "What is clear is that our health is an active state, protected by a series of remarkable defense systems in the body that are firing on all cylinders, from birth to our last day alive, keeping our cells and organs functioning smoothly . . . When you know what to eat to support each health defense, you know how to use your diet to maintain health and beat disease."[6] And, of course, like the United States House of Representatives, all four of us agree that nutrition should be taught in medical school.

The catch? We don't agree on the optimal human diet; more specifically, we don't agree on whether animal foods, whole grains, and fruits should be part of your diet. As you know by now, I believe that all animal foods are destructive to human health, but I fully embrace whole grains and fruits; in fact, I couldn't imagine living without them. Both Dr. Lufkin and Dr. Means renounce grains, although Dr. Means clearly is more skeptical of *refined* grains than whole grains (and perhaps Dr. Lufkin is as well?). Dr. Means permits fruits in the diet, but Dr. Lufkin appears to limit fruits to roughly one a day, and he doesn't even include them in his shopping list of "food groups" for daily consumption. (Dr. Lufkin writes that "In the 1900s, most people consumed about 15 g of fructose a day, usually in a healthy form, such as fruit. That's the equivalent of one piece of fruit or a cup of blueberries. Today, that's nearly quadrupled to 55 g a day, largely from unnatural high fructose corn syrup sources."[7] I agree with his point about excessive fructose consumption, and I take his statement as a clue that he favors no more than one serving of fruit per day.) Dr. Lufkin doesn't say much about nuts, seeds, and legumes in his book, so I'm not sure whether he wants you to eat them; Dr. Means embraces those foods. Dr. Li generally embraces a WPF diet like mine but includes seafood and occasionally, in a very limited way, appears to give the green light to other animal foods.

The disagreements between us on diet raise a sticky wicket that I'll address in this chapter: If we all agree that nutrition should be taught in medical school, but we don't agree on the optimal diet, then exactly *whose* ideas on nutrition should be taught to the doctors of tomorrow?

The opportunity? If we can utilize synergies on the issues on which we *do* agree, and at least find a way forward that provides a process for medical schools to address the aforementioned sticky wicket, we can provide some useful guidance for both our medical community and the population at large.

Of course, I don't mean to suggest that we are the only four doctors whose opinions matter. There are over a million doctors in America, and we are merely four among a million equals. But to a large extent, our ideas represent viewpoints with a growing body of support in the medical community; in my case, I add my voice to the growing chorus of thousands of plant-based physicians and other health professionals who participate in, or support, such organizations as the Plantrician Project, the American College of Lifestyle Medicine, and the Physicians Committee for Responsible Medicine. (Dr. Li would share my enthusiasm for those plant-based organizations, I'm sure, in spite of his acceptance of some animal foods in the diet.) Dr. Lufkin adds his voice to what I might call the ketogenic chorus, emphasizing a high-fat diet that is generally adopted as a high-animal-food diet (although there is such a thing as a vegan keto diet). Dr. Means is something of a maverick who has charted a middle course: She believes that both the whole plant food diet that I advocate and Dr. Lufkin's ketogenic diet can work just fine, as long as the practitioners of those diets avoid processed foods, sugars, and artificial chemicals in their food, while aiming for whole, organic, and even "regenerative" food sources. In short, you might say she cares more about the *quality* of the food you eat than whether it is of animal or plant origin. I'm sure that Dr. Lufkin and Dr. Li would agree with Dr. Means, as I do, that the quality of food matters greatly—and that organically grown produce is always preferable, as it doesn't contain pesticides or other chemical toxins, and it's better for the farmworkers who grow and harvest it—but I chafe at the suggestion that there is any such thing as a high-quality animal food.

I would be remiss not to note that another medical author, Dr. Christopher M. Palmer, a researcher in the field of neuroscience and a practicing psychiatrist, has written a bestselling book concerning mental health, *Brain Energy*, that aligns with the zeitgeist I am describing: The book makes a compelling case that mental diseases are also often the result of metabolic disorders and can be addressed through diet. In Dr. Palmer's words (italics his), "*mental disorders are metabolic disorders of the brain.*"[8] Dr. Palmer does not recommend any specific diet, but I think it's fair to say that he puts the same emphasis on food quality that Dr. Means does, and that he has found particularly good results in some psychiatric cases with use of the ketogenic diet. He also points out that such a high-fat diet could be constructed with a vegan, vegetarian, or omnivorous approach. Since Dr. Palmer does not propose any particular diet, I won't be addressing his ideas further here, except to congratulate him on his valuable contribution in adding mental health to the list of conditions that may hinge on metabolism.

The Ketogenic Diet

Let's take a look first at Dr. Lufkin's ideas, which were shaped by his personal health journey.

Apparently, the doctor used to be slightly overweight, with high blood pressure and prediabetes. He suffered from gout and had a lipid profile that he describes as "alarming."[9]

His recovery from this state involved abstaining from "sugars, processed carbs, processed seed oils, and grains."[10] After transitioning to his new ketogenic diet, he had an experience similar to that of one of the first patients I treated with food therapy: He felt lightheaded when he stood up—the result of the blood pressure medication that he had been taking and that he no longer needed. So, whereas I had helped my patient return to a healthy blood pressure, free of pharmaceutical assistance, by avoiding animal foods and oils, Dr. Lufkin achieved the same result by abstaining from sugars, "processed carbs," and oils.

Exactly what Dr. Lufkin means by "processed carbs" I do not know. Would a blueberry muffin eaten at a diner be one of those "processed carbs"? I'm guessing that's how Dr. Lufkin would label a blueberry muffin, and if I'm right about that, such a label would not be without some justification. The diner's blueberry muffin would surely contain a lot of sugar, and it would also contain some form of flour, probably white flour—these are indeed "processed carbs" (in the case of sugar, it's pure carbohydrate). The muffin would likely also contain oil, and possibly butter, and possibly eggs—but these are not carbs; they are high-fat foods. So it might be just as accurate to call the muffin a "processed fat" as a "processed carb." Hopefully, the muffin would also contain blueberries; these are not processed carbs, but whole fruits, although baking them is not the most healthful way to eat them.

In short, I would argue that that blueberry muffin is unhealthy not only because of its sugar content but also because of the fat. The flour is no health bargain, either; the more refined, the more inflammatory it will be. The blueberries are good for you, naturally, but they'd be healthier still eaten raw. So if Dr. Lufkin's former diet involved a daily blueberry muffin from the local diner, and his new, improved diet eliminated that muffin, then it's not surprising to me that his health improved. But it would be not only because he eliminated some unhealthy refined carbs but also because he eliminated some oil and other unhealthy fats.

Dr. Lufkin's lipids also improved, he maintains, on the ketogenic diet. He writes that his triglycerides lowered and his "good cholesterol" (HDL cholesterol) increased. (He doesn't mention what happened to his total serum cholesterol numbers or his LDL cholesterol levels.)

A word about HDL cholesterol: It is somewhat overrated and misunderstood as a health metric. A person can be perfectly healthy with a low HDL score, especially if that person has low serum cholesterol. Drugs designed to increase the HDL level in the blood have achieved that end effectively—without in any way reducing heart attacks or strokes, which was, of course, the whole point of developing them.[11] Think of HDL cholesterol as the "garbage trucks" that come and escort away the "garbage" (cholesterol molecules) to the liver for excretion ("reverse cholesterol transport"). If you have less garbage, you require fewer garbage trucks. HDL cholesterol and total serum cholesterol therefore often (but not always) move in tandem, and when they do so, in most circumstances I would rather see a patient's serum cholesterol and HDL cholesterol both *decrease* than both *increase*, given that choice.

Dr. Lufkin's insulin resistance also resolved, he believes, and his gout disappeared. His improved health achieved on the keto diet inspired him with a determination to encourage others to experience that way of eating, and he did so not only by writing *Lies I Taught in Medical School* but also with other initiatives, such as attempting to create graduate medical training programs.

I can readily believe that Dr. Lufkin's health improved in exactly the ways he reports. Remember, at the same time that he was starting on the keto diet, he was very helpfully giving up "sweets, baked goods, and processed foods."[12] He was also apparently skipping breakfast and lunch, meaning that he was practicing intermittent fasting to a very effective degree. There were two fewer meals a day at which he could eat anything harmful, and presumably his overall calorie intake went down. The problem is that if, like Dr. Lufkin, you eat hardly any carbohydrates but continue to consume a high-fat diet that clogs up your insulin receptor function, you can generate insulin resistance but never know it, because you never experience its effects. That is, you're not eating the carbohydrates that would otherwise liberate the simple sugars that you would have trouble metabolizing, and that would stay in your bloodstream.

We each have our own health stories. My story, as you know, is that I lost weight, improved my blood pressure and my blood sugar levels, and became much healthier on a WPF diet. Dr. Lufkin lost weight and got healthier on the regimen described above. Dr. Means writes that she achieved excellent health and resolved her own serious digestive troubles both on a vegan whole foods diet and also on a diet incorporating animal foods. All three of us overcame vexing health issues. I can believe everyone's story, but all of our stories amount to just anecdotes.

As relevant as they may be to our private perspectives on health, we need to put our personal anecdotes aside and focus on the science. The question for Dr. Lufkin is: What are the long-term effects of eating a diet that is 60 to 80 percent fat? That is generally recognized as the proportion of fat required in the diet in order that people can attain ketosis, the state he favors as a kind of ongoing metabolic lifestyle, in which fat is metabolized as a primary fuel. Has any population in human history ever kept up a diet like that? You might think that the Inuits, with limited access to plant food, have existed in a ketogenic state, but studies indicate that is not the case.[13] In any case, Inuit longevity is not impressive.[14]

Let me be clear: There is a role for ketosis. If you engage in the healthy practice of intermittent fasting, in which you allow your digestive system to rest from the evening until, say, the late morning, ingesting no food for fourteen to sixteen hours, your body may begin to activate the process of ketosis and you may burn some fat as fuel. That's a good thing. If you undertake a medically supervised water fast and eat no food for several days, your body will surely go into ketosis, and you may lose some visceral fat, leading sometimes to dramatic health improvements, such as lower blood pressure and reduced inflammation. That's a good thing, and ketosis is what makes it happen. A ketogenic diet has also been demonstrated to reduce seizures in some people with epilepsy. But that does not mean that ketosis should be the state that all of us should aspire to achieve and maintain 24/7, or that there's anything risky about metabolizing the primary fuel for the human body, which is carbohydrates.

By contrast, there likely are some definite risks to staying in ketosis in the long term:

1. **Increased risk of nutrient deficiencies.** Since ketogenic diets often exclude or severely limit fruits, whole grains, and legumes, which are rich in essential vitamins, minerals, and fiber, this can lead to deficiencies in vitamin C, folate, magnesium, and potassium—all needed for immune function, heart health, and cellular metabolism.[15]
2. **Potential cardiovascular risks.** While some short-term studies suggest ketogenic diets may improve certain cardiovascular markers, such as triglycerides, long-term adherence may raise atherogenic LDL due to the high intake of saturated fats, increasing the risk for heart disease and generalized atherosclerosis.[16]
3. The **high protein content** of meat-based, ketogenic diets can strain and even damage kidney filters (glomeruli) and also lead to kidney stone formation. This diet could be patently unsafe for someone with preexisting but undiagnosed kidney disease.[17]
4. **Increased risk of osteoporosis.** Long-term ketosis can lead to bone mineral loss due to chronic acidosis and the leaching of calcium from bones, leading to decreased bone density and increased fracture risk over time.[18]
5. **Adverse gut microbiome changes.** Ketogenic diets tend to be low in dietary fiber, which is essential for gut microbiota diversity, leading to gut dysbiosis, constipation, and an increased risk of colon cancer due to lack of short-chain fatty acid production.[19]
6. **Impaired glucose metabolism and insulin resistance.** While ketogenic diets can initially lower blood sugar, prolonged ketosis may impair the body's ability to handle carbohydrates efficiently, with some individuals developing physiologic insulin resistance as the dietary fats pile up in the muscle cells as intramyocellular lipid and inhibit insulin receptors. This may make it harder to tolerate even small amounts of carbohydrates in the long run.[20]
7. **Cognitive and mental health concerns.** While some individuals report improved mental clarity on ketogenic diets, long-term

ketosis can deplete serotonin precursors and impair neurotransmitter balance, potentially contributing to mood swings, depression, and anxiety.[21]

8. **Increased all-cause mortality.** Large epidemiological studies have associated animal-food-based, low-carbohydrate, high-fat diets with increased all-cause mortality rates.[22]

It is hard to see this dietary approach as sustainable, safe, or smart for long-term nutrition.

Like Gary Taubes and other keto advocates and authors, Dr. Lufkin expresses his low opinion of "carbohydrates." The whole thesis of the keto diet is to almost completely eliminate "carbohydrates" in the diet.

I put the word in quotes because it's not easy for me to grasp what Dr. Lufkin and his ketogenic colleagues mean by "carbohydrates." Or why he insists on conflating healthy foods that (like most healthy foods) happen to be rich in carbohydrates—fruits, vegetables, whole grains, legumes—with processed foods high in sugar (a can of soda, say), labeling them all "carbs." He allows vegetables on his proposed diet, but fruits are mostly shunned and whole grains get banned as "carbohydrates," even though they also contain protein and fat. A can of soda is not cousin to a head of broccoli or a fresh mango, and the same term ("carbs") should not be used to refer to all.

Dr. Lufkin argues that good health is conferred by eating six sources of food: eggs, meat, chicken, fish, vegetables, and cheese. That is the "shopping list" he recommends.[23] Five of these six acceptable food sources are animal foods, all high in fat, including heart disease–promoting saturated fat and cholesterol. Only one of his six acceptable food sources contains fiber: vegetables. Only one of his acceptable food sources contains significant antioxidant content: again, vegetables. Only one of his acceptable food sources is proven to boast anti-inflammatory properties: once again, vegetables. I'm not sure how Dr. Lufkin feels about nuts and seeds—you'd think he might favor them because they are fatty, but they are omitted from his list. Nor do I know where he stands on legumes, but since they are not fatty, and they're not on his shopping list, I'm deducing that he would minimize or eliminate them. I'll note that author Dan Buettner's study of the longest-living and healthiest global human populations demonstrated that beans are the food staple that recur in those "Blue Zones" around the world. But despite that pedigree, beans are not fatty, so they can't be particularly welcome on a ketogenic diet.

The ketogenic diet all but forces its practitioners to obsess over macronutrients in a desperate (and, I would argue, generally doomed) attempt to eat fat and more fat, while shunning carbohydrates. In my view, that's neither a nourishing way to eat nor a fulfilling way to live. When I open my pantry, I don't see a big macronutrient box labeled FATS, another box labeled CARBOHYDRATES, and a third labeled PROTEINS. Instead, I might see, for example, a bag of rolled oats. Well, the caloric content of oatmeal breaks down roughly this way: about 77 percent carbohydrate, about 15 percent protein, about 8 percent fat. If I were to store my food in macronutrient boxes, which one should I put my rolled oats in? I have no idea.

I also have different types of beans and lentils in my pantry. Kidney beans, for example, derive about 70 percent of their calories from carbohydrate, about 27 percent of their calories from protein, and about 3 percent of their calories from fat. Which macronutrient box should I store my kidney beans in? Beats me.

I also have some lightly processed foods in my pantry. I have a jar of tomato sauce, for example. It's made from organic tomatoes, organic onions, organic garlic, organic basil, and organic spices. Which macronutrient box does that go in?

In short, I don't store *macronutrients* in my pantry; I store *food*. Whole foods for humans (i.e., unprocessed plant foods) always contain a component of all the macronutrients, and whole foods always contain fiber, which can be thought of as a kind of calorie-free form of carbohydrate. To linguistically reduce foods to single macronutrients makes no scientific sense, although it's a favorite parlor trick of diet book authors. Don't let anyone fool you into believing that potatoes are "carbs"; that is a reductive and unhelpful way of viewing a marvelous food. Potatoes are root vegetables that contain a healthy amount of protein and a smidgen of fat along with carbohydrate, fiber, water, and micronutrients. Similarly, meat is not "protein"; meat is the decaying muscle tissue of an animal, and it usually contains roughly as many calories from fat as from protein. Much of the fat in meat will be dangerous saturated fat, and an additional small portion of it will be naturally occurring and even more dangerous trans-fat. It would certainly make as much sense, therefore, to call meat a "fat" as to call it a "protein," but try explaining that to your waiter. In any case, the public relations teams in the animal foods industry are united in their determination to sell meat as a "protein," not a "fat"—the reality that it contains excessive amounts of both be damned. They know very well that it would be harder to fool people into believing that they can build up their muscles by eating a lot of fat.

Dr. Lufkin is not specific about what percentage of your calories he wants you to ingest as fat, but again, since he clearly endorses the ketogenic diet, and therefore wants your diet to induce ketosis, I have to assume that he wants you to ingest at least 60 percent, and perhaps even as much as 80 percent, of calories as fat. Just think about what that means. All the items in my pantry—the oats, the kidney beans, the tomato sauce, and frankly everything else except the nuts and seeds—will be way too low in fat to help you achieve ketosis. So if you go wild and have a single serving of kidney beans in tomato sauce, for example, you'll have to quickly compensate for that indulgent straying from the keto path, and for the rest of the day you'll need to limit yourself to foods that are *even more fatty* than the already obscenely fatty overall objective of the diet. You'll run into that same dilemma if you are decadent enough to eat an apple, or a banana, or too many vegetables, or a slice of bread, or even if you make the mistake of eating some animal foods that are not fatty, such as shrimp or egg whites.

The fatty animal foods on Dr. Lufkin's shopping list will be almost completely devoid of antioxidants, so a ketogenic diet forfeits your best opportunity to fortify yourself against cancer and other diseases.

Dr. Lufkin's book makes a strong case against sugar and particularly fructose, but nowhere within it do I find a word against the WPF diet or a refutation of its capacity to help you reach the same ends he has achieved: healthfully low blood pressure, stable blood glucose, clean arteries, and a healthy heart. In fact, concerning the two macronutrients—fats and proteins—that he considers (in a barbed slap at carbohydrates) "essential," he writes: "You can get all your fats and proteins from plant sources, such as avocados and beans, for instance, without relying on animal products such as meat, dairy, or eggs, at which point your diet is what we would call a *vegan diet*."[24] He also writes, "I believe that almost any nutrition style from vegan to carnivore can be healthy if done properly. This means avoiding processed foods, which will make any diet unhealthy."[25]

This leads me to wonder: If, even according to Dr. Lufkin, any nutrition style, including vegan, can be healthy, then why eat a fiber-deficient diet in which you have to be afraid of a piece of fruit, an ear of corn, or a bean burrito when you can achieve the same—and I would argue far greater—health benefits on a WPF diet that does not require the killing of animals, the razing of forests for grazing land, the disregard for our place in evolution as a herbivorous primate, or a constant obsession with macronutrient content as you struggle mightily to hit your daily fat goal?

In his book's "Closing Thoughts," Dr. Lufkin laments that "A typical cardiologist might still suggest that an at-risk patient eat low-fat, high-sugar foods, for example."[26] Well, I *do* know some cardiologists—the better ones—who recommend a low-fat diet to their at-risk patients. As we have seen, Dr. Esselstyn achieved health outcomes that were extraordinary and unprecedented by enrolling his very-high-risk patients on a low-fat diet exclusively composed of plant foods. But are there cardiologists who recommend "high-sugar foods" to their patients? Here Dr. Lufkin creates confusion by allowing the reader to conflate refined sugar and sweeteners—which surely all good cardiologists counsel against—with the natural sugars in fruit, and perhaps with foods that are high in starch, such as potatoes, sweet potatoes, corn, beans, and rice. Our bodies will then convert the starch to glucose at a controlled rate. That does not make a sweet potato a "high-sugar food" that threatens your heart.

In another of Dr. Lufkin's closing thoughts, he contends that it is a lie that "All dietary cholesterol is bad for you."[27] Well, like all vegans, I eat a diet that contains zero dietary cholesterol, and I have done so for the last four decades. My liver functions as all livers do, providing for my body all the vital cholesterol that it needs. If it's a lie that "all dietary cholesterol is bad for you," then it would likely follow that "some dietary cholesterol is good for you." For what purpose, exactly? Clearly, I haven't needed it. Nor has any vegan friend or patient I've ever encountered suffered any health slight from their lack of dietary cholesterol. We know perfectly well that there is no need for dietary cholesterol, and given the well-established link between dietary cholesterol and heart disease, I think it is indeed safe and accurate to posit that "all dietary cholesterol is bad for you." It's a truth, I would argue, not a lie.

Can All Diets Work?

Dr. Means, who was nominated for US surgeon general in 2025 (although that nomination appears to be stalled at this writing in part because of an inactive medical license), is a woman of formidable intellect whose book *Good Energy* addresses not only diet but also any number of lifestyle issues affecting health: timing your meals, eating mindfully, practicing breathwork, walking after eating, promoting sleep by avoiding the use of artificial light at night and creating a dark and quiet bedroom, spending time outdoors, protecting your circadian rhythm, making use of standing desks, understanding the value of heat exposure and cold exposure, avoiding plastics, avoiding scented products, cultivating a sense of community, and more. Kudos to Dr. Means for delineating many of the innumerable factors beyond diet that may play a significant role in your physical well-being, your happiness, and your lifespan. It may well be the case that nobody has brought all those factors together between book covers in a more comprehensive way than she has.

The title *Good Energy* serves as a unifying principle for the book's many subjects. Implicitly, she's saying that it is not only good food that can bestow "good energy" through healthful metabolism, but deep sleep, sunshine, and caring friends can help do so, as well. Bravo, I say.

My only significant disagreement with Dr. Means concerns diet, and here that disagreement is nuanced because I don't think that she would in any way find fault with my own WPF diet. Dr. Means makes her position on diet abundantly clear in the middle of her book:

> I personally know brilliant, hardworking, highly educated people who believe polar opposite ideologies about nutrition. One group feels that a low-fat, high-carb diet is the only diet that yields Good Energy, and another feels that a high-fat, low-carb diet is the best way. Both have data that show that these diets reduce liver fat (a key marker of insulin sensitivity), lower weight, lower triglycerides, improve insulin sensitivity, and lower inflammation. And both are right. And in between is the Mediterranean diet, which also has masses of literature to support a more omnivorous approach. All these diets can "work" for good health because *all* emphasize primarily unprocessed, whole foods to give the cells what they need to function and cue satiety mechanisms so that we don't overeat.[28]

Thus, from Dr. Means's point of view, both Dr. Lufkin, who believes that the six basic food groups from which you should feed yourself are eggs, meat, chicken, fish, vegetables, and cheese, and I, who believe that the five basic food groups from which you should feed yourself are fruits, vegetables, whole grains, legumes, and nuts and seeds, are right, even though the only type of food for which we seem to share enthusiasm is vegetables—and, given Dr. Lufkin's severe requirement of a diet fatty enough to induce ketosis, I doubt that his diet would accommodate as many vegetables as mine. While Dr. Lufkin and I stand mercifully in agreement on the salubrity of vegetables, I believe that his entire larder of eggs, meat, chicken, fish, and cheese should be shunned, as all these foods will increase your risk of obesity, high blood pressure, type 2 diabetes, and heart disease, with the fish posing an additional risk of neurological disease. I'll let Dr. Lufkin speak for himself on any risks he may find in fruits, whole grains, legumes, and nuts and seeds, but it's quite possible that he would be as wary of my shopping list as I am of his.

Yet we're both right, according to Dr. Means. Both diets will work fine, she argues, as long as the foods involved are unprocessed and "sustainably sourced."[29]

"I am so grateful that I have had a foot in both worlds," Dr. Means writes, referring to the vegan world and the "ketogenic and animal-based crowd."[30] She laments the social media posts from vegans that blame carnivores for "ruining the planet," and she considers the "vitriol from the ketogenic and animal-based crowd towards the vegans . . . some of the cruelest stuff I've seen on the internet."[31] She wants us to appreciate that both diets can work and doesn't consider her own position "wishy-washy."[32]

Instead, she seems to believe that human cells will metabolize the muscle meat from the hind end of a pig just as well as they will metabolize a cup of blueberries, as long as the pig was raised on a regenerative farm, and the blueberries were organically grown in healthy soil. She dismisses the risk that ketogenic dieters will be fiber deficient, instead holding out hope that ketogenic dieters may be able, in their own livers, to synthesize butyrate (a most helpful short-chain fatty acid linked to many health benefits, including improved mood), since they likely will lack enough fiber in their gut to ferment into butyrate—the normal route by which those of us who eat a diet rich in plant foods do it.

Butyrate production is not, however, the only basis on which a mountain of scientific evidence proclaims the benefits of fiber. Dr. Means does not address, for example, the risk that a fiber-deficient diet may lead to colon cancer. The ketogenic diet is so wildly unnatural and difficult to sustain that Dr. Means does her readers no favors by straining to find some mechanism by which it could possibly work.

To state what should be obvious, your body will experience a huge contrast between ingesting a cup of blueberries and the hind end of a pig. Do not sell your body short—it can and will readily tell the difference. The blueberries will flood your tissues with anthocyanins and other antioxidants and phytochemicals that will do nothing but nourish and protect you. The hind end of a pig will cause inflammation because it is decaying flesh, rife with bacteria and endotoxins, that offers no nutrients that you can't obtain in better form from plant foods. Animal protein is excessive in its concentration and is carcinogenic, and there's no good reason to believe that pig fat will do anything for you other than make you fat and help to clog your arteries.

Your body will react in profoundly different ways to a ketogenic diet that is 60 to 80 percent fat and a WPF diet that is 10 to 20 percent fat. By shrugging at this difference and promising that, as long as the fat is from the butter of organically raised cows or the lard of regeneratively raised pigs, your body will barely register the difference, Dr. Means is not, as she wishes, escaping polarizing nutritional ideologies. Instead, she's creating a peculiar kind of ideology of her own: blind nutritional neutrality.

I do not know or understand the scientific basis on which Dr. Means assumes her neutral position on plant foods versus animal foods. Since she has a prodigious intellect, I can't dismiss her as simply being conflict averse. But, to me, it is nothing short of bizarre to try to make the case that it makes no metabolic difference whether you ingest blueberries or pig.

Planetary Health vs. Personal Health

Gary Taubes, a journalist who may be the most notable keto diet advocate in the country, wrote these words in *The Wall Street Journal*:

> Choosing to avoid meat and eat a plant-based diet has never seemed so virtuous and necessary. Between the intrinsic cruelty of industrial livestock production and livestock's climate footprint—estimated by the U.N.'s Food and Agriculture Organization to be 14.5% of all greenhouse gases world-wide, significantly greater than that of plant agriculture—it has become increasingly difficult to defend the place of meat and animal-sourced foods in our diets.[33]

Taubes nonetheless goes on to make the case that, at least for "those predisposed to become obese and/or diabetic, carbohydrate-rich foods trigger that predisposition,"[34] and that a ketogenic diet saves such people from obesity or type 2 diabetes. He believes that insulin is secreted in response to carbohydrates, whether from fruit, legumes, or starches, and that fat storage thereby increases. Thus, he blames obesity on the proposition that carbohydrates "have some unique ability to stimulate fat accumulation."[35]

I believe that Taubes is very wrong about almost all of that, and, as with Dr. Lufkin and other keto diet advocates, I find his use of the term "carbohydrates" confusing, but I admire his intellectual honesty in acknowledging that the animal-based diet that he practices and commends to others presents a threat to planetary well-being. He acknowledges that a ketogenic diet can be constructed from fatty plant foods but worries that, "as with any eating pattern, the degree to which people enjoy the recommended foods has a strong bearing on whether they will stick to them. For many people, meat and meat-based foods provide satisfactions that plants cannot. So the tension remains: The healthiest diet for those predisposed to become fat and diabetic may not be what's healthiest for the planet."[36]

His conclusion may be less than stirring but still remains intellectually consistent: "no one can tell us whether we should subordinate our own health and well-being—and perhaps that of our children too—to that of the planet. That is a personal decision. If that trade-off is the reality of our food situation in the century ahead, we have to accept the consequences when we make our choices."[37]

Of course, it's my opinion that we humans actually stand in a far more fortunate position: I believe there is no trade-off at all between our personal health and planetary health, because I see the WPF diet as a boon to both. But I have to accept that Taubes does not agree. He suspects that the WPF diet will make some people—those "predisposed to become fat and diabetic"—well, fat and diabetic. I can say that I have never seen that happen in the forty years that I have advocated this way of eating and instructed patients in following it, but his opinion remains his opinion. I have, of course, indeed seen vegans who eat too much in the way of processed food, sugary treats, and oils gain weight, and I suspect that Taubes confuses such vegans with those on the WPF diet.

Has the proportion of people with awful genes that make them "predisposed to become fat and diabetic" skyrocketed in recent decades along with our rates of obesity and diabetes, I wonder, or could the problem possibly be not their genes but what they've been eating? The percentage of the population eating the WPF diet is unfortunately minuscule, perhaps 1 percent, so with the population of those overweight or obese standing at 73 percent, it would be a little rich to blame the increase in obesity on us.

Taubes clearly wrestles with the conflict between planetary health and what he believes to be the most practical diet for weight loss (a fatty, meat-based diet). Perhaps if I could introduce him to the thousands of people who have overcome overweight, obesity, and even morbid obesity on the planet-friendly WPF diet, his concerns would be allayed.

Dr. Means, unlike Taubes, believes that the WPF diet works quite well while also believing that the ketogenic program of Dr. Lufkin and Taubes can work quite well. And Dr. Lufkin himself, as we know, has acknowledged that "almost any nutrition style from vegan to carnivore can be healthy if done properly."[38] This raises the question: If you believe that both diets work just fine, why wouldn't you endorse the diet that can save the planet instead of the diet that wreaks havoc on it? Why wouldn't you share Taubes's concerns for the environment? Why would you fail to even note that one diet requires the suffering of billions of sentient creatures, and the other does not? If you believe that the health outcomes of these opposing diets are effectively a wash, why not insist that the environmental and moral consequences of these diets come into play?

If we are meant to buy into the contention—as I readily do—that chronic stress, lack of sunlight, unhealthy sleep patterns, and overuse of artificial light can create "Bad Energy," shouldn't we ask ourselves if confining animals to crates and obscenely crowded warehouses in which they fester in their own waste for their short, miserable lifetimes before they are slaughtered might do the same—to both the animals so treated and the humans who consume their flesh? What about the Bad Energy caused by food poisoning from the enteric bacteria in slaughterhouses and in animal waste sprayed on farms? Why not endorse the diet that can prevent pandemics—sources of boundless Bad Energy—instead of the diet that will create them?

I suspect that Dr. Means would have a ready answer to these criticisms: She would say that, indeed, she opposes CAFOs (concentrated animal feeding operations) and endorses only meat that is grass fed, poultry that is pasture raised or free range, and free-range pork. She would consider those animals humanely raised. I would note that another popular diet book author, Dr. Mark Hyman, takes that exact position in his book *The Pegan Diet*: He wants you to eat meat but only if it's regeneratively raised. In his words, "You are not what you eat; you are whatever you are eating has eaten."[39] That strikes me as an attenuated dietary philosophy; we all certainly have more control over what we eat than over our food's food. And we gain nothing by cycling our nutrients through animals. Dr. Hyman does not believe that conventionally raised meat is healthy, but he *does* think that regeneratively raised meat is healthy: "After decades of reviewing the science, it is clear that grass-fed, regeneratively raised meat, cooked in the right way and combined with medicinal spices in the context of a plant-rich, whole foods, unprocessed diet, is not only not bad for your health—it might be beneficial . . ."[40]

Unfortunately, the "organic," "grass-fed," "pasture-raised," "free-range," and "regeneratively raised" animals tend to be killed in the same slaughterhouses as the CAFO animals. Slaughterhouses rank as simply the most miserable working environments that you will find in this country, and the meatpacking industry is perennially notorious for its despicable practice of employing undocumented child labor in highly dangerous work.[41] While in theory the pasture-raised animals will arrive at the slaughterhouse in a separate shipment from the CAFO animals, I would not blindly trust that industry to meticulously segregate the regeneratively raised animals from the animals that were not so "lucky." The regeneratively raised animals will in any case generate the same fear hormones as the CAFO animals when they are shipped to, and when they enter, that same slaughterhouse, and count me as highly skeptical that there would be any significant health difference between eating the flesh of a grass-fed bovine and the flesh of a CAFO bovine. That's a thin reed indeed on which to bet one's health.

One study compared young women who ate a diet of pasture-fed beef and dairy products (the "CLA diet," a reference to conjugated linoleic acid, assumed to be higher in pasture-fed beef and dairy) with young women who ate those products from grain-fed cattle, for a period of almost two months. The study's authors concluded: "The CLA diet did not result in any differences in insulin sensitivity, body composition, circulating blood lipids, or other measured disease risk factors as compared with the control diet. Thus, we conclude that a diet naturally enriched with over a 3-fold increase in CLA from pasture-fed cattle did not significantly alter selected health risk factors in healthy, premenopausal women as compared with a similar diet composed of foods from grain-fed cattle."[42]

I would love to conduct an experiment in which two steaks are given each to Dr. Hyman and Dr. Means. They have to decide which was pasture raised and which was CAFO raised. I don't believe they'd be able to determine the answer by look, smell, or taste. I don't believe they'd be able to determine the answer by how they felt after eating. And I don't believe they'd be able to determine the answer if they dissected the steaks and examined them under a microscope. But they are able to make their assertion of the superiority of "grass-fed," "organic," or "regenerative" meat safe in the knowledge that nobody will challenge them. They are thereby able to position themselves as doctors with a moderate, sensible, balanced approach to nutrition who are not asking Americans to give up their cherished flesh foods, while they still condemn industrial animal agriculture, an enterprise that is widely unpopular.

I would estimate that the number of meat-eating Americans who meticulously limit themselves to only regeneratively raised meat would be smaller even than those who eat the WPF diet. When was the last time you heard anyone in a high-end steakhouse order a filet mignon, but only after insisting that it must be regeneratively raised? Does anyone ordering a burger in a fast-food joint require that it be organic and grass fed? Does anyone in any restaurant insist that their regeneratively raised meat not be cooked at high temperatures, as Dr. Hyman recommends, because, as he rightly acknowledges, "High-temperature cooking or grilling (veggies or meat) produces toxic compounds, including heterocyclic amines, polycyclic aromatic hydrocarbons, and advanced glycation end products (AGEs), which can damage your arteries and cause cancer"?[43] Or insist that the chef cook the regeneratively raised meat with a sufficient amount of spices, as Dr. Hyman recommends, to protect you from inflammation? This "regeneratively raised" nonsense is not a real, substantial movement meant to save anyone's health or the environment; it is simply an intellectual talking point for health influencers who want to sidestep the grim realities that animal agriculture presents us with.

Dr. Hyman acknowledges that the labeling of poultry products is "confusing" and mostly "meaningless,"[44] and that the label "free-range" "does not require any designated amount of time that the birds can roam, and it does not tell us about the birds' diet."[45] We also have to keep in mind that chickens that are "pasture-raised" or "free-range" are not given rides to the slaughterhouse in an Uber. They arrive in the same cramped trucks as chickens that spent their whole short lives crammed into warehouses. They are not provided with food or water during the journey. Any distinction that may exist between the fates of the "pasture-raised" and industrially farmed animals fades into oblivion on the last day of their lives.

As PETA (People for the Ethical Treatment of Animals) reports, "Cows on organic dairy farms can be kept in crowded sheds, mired in their own waste, much like cows on factory dairy farms. They, too, are artificially impregnated every year, and their calves are taken from them soon after birth. Cows on organic farms often aren't given antibiotics—even when they're sick or when their udders become infected, something that happens often—because medicated animals lose their 'organic' status."[46] At peta.org, you will find photo and video evidence of shocking, chilling animal cruelty, even at farms advertised as "humane."

Would Dr. Means approve of "free-range eggs" raised by a company with "organics" in its name, especially if those eggs were advertised as coming from hens that "can peck, perch, and play on plenty of green grass"?[47] I suspect she might be inclined to do so. Unfortunately, there have been multiple lawsuits about deceptive advertising in the egg industry. The company that made that sweet claim about its playful hens housed them, according to the plaintiffs, twenty thousand strong, in warehouses for most of their lives. The company defended its marketing as merely a "whimsical description of what chickens do in grass"[48]—before settling the lawsuit. I would ask Dr. Means: Given the track record of animal agriculture interests, why should anyone believe the terms "free-range" or "cage-free" or "pasture-raised," much less believe that it will make any difference in the quality of the food they eat?

Beyond the "greenwashing" of animal cruelty, though, there is the preposterous impracticality of the "humane meat" movement. Dr. Means and Dr. Hyman make the same case that CAFO meat is bad for you while regeneratively raised meat is good for you. They present this case as black and white, but the reality is that most cows are grass fed for at least part of their lives; still, in the US, about 99 percent are "finished" at CAFOs, to which Dr. Means and Dr. Hyman object. Their objection to CAFO products, combined with their embrace of "regenerative" products, creates an elitist fantasy, because if Americans were to continue to eat the same amount of meat that they do now, but eat only purely grass-fed meat, we would need a few new planets to provide all the land that would be required.

While CAFOs are an environmental nightmare, grass-fed meat may actually be worse for the environment, as it's the grazing operations that are responsible for most of the deforestation attendant to animal agriculture; it's the grazing operations that are reducing our soil to dust and creating deserts; it's the grazing operations that are responsible for the lion's share of our biodiversity loss. If Americans are going to continue to eat meat in the massive quantities they do now (not to mention the even greater quantities that Dr. Lufkin would apparently encourage), there never will be any way to accommodate that demand other than with CAFOs, and CAFOs will forever mar our landscape, our waterways, and our air—until we perish.

So even if you are one of the rare meat eaters who proudly consumes only expensive, regeneratively raised bison purchased at Whole Foods, you need to understand that if every meat eater in the country followed in your footsteps, while continuing to consume the same amount of meat as they do now, there would be no land left even for your Whole Foods. It's a pipe dream to imagine that "sustainably raised" meat would be in any way sustainable if everybody ate it. It's only because less than 1 percent of meat-eating Americans even sample it that the fantasy, and the greenwashing, can endure.

The Best Defense

Dr. Li organizes his marvelous book *Eat to Beat Disease* around the premise that there are five natural defense systems of the body: angiogenesis, regeneration, microbiome, DNA protection, and immunity. He trains his focus on which foods to eat to fortify each of these natural defense systems. What a brilliant and original way to contemplate, and activate, the power of nutrition!

Angiogenesis, the body's process of building new blood vessels, can sometimes be a positive and sometimes be a negative. It's a positive when we're talking about increasing blood flow to the heart to combat ischemic heart disease or to the genitals to reverse erectile dysfunction; it's a negative, for example, with cancers, in which increased blood flow to tumors helps them grow, and with age-related macular degeneration, in which abnormal growth of blood vessels causes leaking of fluid beneath the macula (part of the retina at the back of the eye, crucial to vision). So angiogenesis needs to be kept in balance.

Dr. Li points out that soy foods do just that, combatting both diseases of excessive angiogenesis like cancer and diseases of insufficient angiogenesis like heart disease.[49] Tomatoes, which can inhibit angiogenesis, have been demonstrated to help prevent prostate cancer.[50] The good news, according to Dr. Li, is that "foods cannot override the body's own natural set points for angiogenesis. This means that anti-angiogenic foods can't reduce the number of blood vessels in the body needed to maintain the health of your organs. And it also means that angiogenesis-stimulating foods can't shut down your body's defensive ability to keep excessive blood vessels pruned back so they cannot cause disease."[51]

So what foods does Dr. Li recommend to promote healthy angiogenesis balance? Besides soy and tomatoes, the list is long and includes cruciferous vegetables (broccoli, bok choy, cauliflower, kale, and more); stone fruit (peaches, plums, nectarines, apricots, cherries, and more); apples; berries (strawberries, raspberries, blackberries, blueberries, and cranberries); many teas; tree nuts, including walnuts, pecans, almonds, cashews, pistachios, pine nuts, and macadamia nuts; cocoa powder; and such spices as rosemary, oregano, turmeric, licorice, and cinnamon.[52] All these plant foods are believed to be helpful because of their role in controlling angiogenesis and promoting its proper balance. Then there are the foods that Dr. Li informs us will stimulate angiogenesis in a helpful way: barley; seeds such as flaxseed, sunflower seeds, sesame seeds, pumpkin seeds, and chia seeds; and foods containing ursolic acid (ginseng, rosemary, peppermint, apple peel, and dried fruits).[53] Foods containing quercetin have been proven to both stimulate angiogenesis "in the face of oxygen deprivation of tissues"[54] and inhibit tumor angiogenesis, thus making these foods ideal for angiogenesis balance. Dr. Li's list of quercetin-rich foods includes capers, onions, red-leaf lettuce, hot green chile peppers, cranberries, black plums, and apples.[55]

While all of Dr. Li's suggested foods to stimulate angiogenesis are plant based, he does include a number of animal foods in his list of beneficially anti-angiogenic foods, and these include some types of fish and some types of cheese. Without debating these foods' capacity to contribute to angiogenesis balance, I would simply say that if the goal is to eat foods that may help prevent or control cancer, it makes no sense to eat cheese, which contains cancer-promoting casein and introduces to your body insulin-like growth factor 1 (IGF-1), which has been linked to cancer growth;[56] fish consumption, meanwhile, has been associated with melanoma[57] and, as discussed earlier, with neurological disease. Both cheese and fish will of course also contribute saturated fat and cholesterol to your bloodstream, without fiber. In short, why not choose from the long list of plant foods that promote angiogenesis balance, as well as provide many other benefits, without the downsides?

Regeneration refers to the body's capacity to use stem cells to rebuild and renew tissues. Dr. Li explains in detail how stem cells can be damaged by such conditions as type 2 diabetes;[58] therefore, the trick is to eat the diet that boosts stem cells before they get too badly damaged. At the same time, to prevent that damage, you may need to ditch the diet you are eating, or the alcohol you may be drinking, or the cigarettes you may be smoking.

Most of the many foods that Dr. Li suggests to promote regeneration are plant foods: green beans, black chokeberries, black raspberries, goji berries, rice bran, turmeric, mangoes, green tea, and black tea.[59] The only exceptions are two food sources from the sea (squid ink and fish oil), which can be laden with contaminants. Again, I reveal my bias that all foods from the sea should be avoided, in your own best interest and in the best interest of our fragile, overfished oceans.

Dr. Li's recommended foods for the microbiome again skew heavily towards the plant side of the equation, unsurprisingly: pumpernickel bread, kiwifruit, bamboo shoots, beans, walnuts, mushrooms, broccoli, cauliflower, bok choy, and other brassica vegetables.[60] He also believes that some dairy foods, such as yogurt and Camembert cheese, can serve as probiotic foods. However, I'd humbly suggest that you get your probiotics without the saturated fat and *with* the fiber.

One way DNA defends our health, Dr. Li points out, is by protecting itself through the mechanism of DNA self-repair. This amazing molecule can control epigenetic change, which can be thought of as turning on or off some of the many genes that reside on the DNA strand; epigenetics, then, is our capacity to either suppress or activate our genes. Telomeres, repetitive DNA sequences at the end of chromosomes—think of the aglet caps at the end of shoelaces—protect our DNA, with longer telomeres predictive of longer lifespans. Dr. Li's champion foods for promoting DNA repair are antioxidant-rich foods, such as berry juices (or simply berries), kiwifruit, carrots, broccoli, and lycopene-rich foods such as tomato, watermelon, guava, and pink grapefruit.[61] For epigenetic support, he recommends turning to soy, cruciferous vegetables, coffee, tea, and turmeric.[62] For telomere protection, Dr. Li would have you look to coffee again, tea, nuts and seeds, and a vegetable-rich diet. At the same time, to protect against DNA damage, Dr. Li cautions against fatty foods, processed meat, and sugar-sweetened beverages.[63] To be fully transparent, Dr. Li also finds DNA protection stemming from oysters and seafood, but since these foods also carry neurological risks and a long list of contaminants, and since we need to protect not only our DNA but also our oceans, why not get all your DNA protection from the long list of plant foods that Dr. Li puts forth?

To enhance your body's immune system, Dr. Li touts the benefits of a long list of fruits and vegetables and mushrooms. He has only one animal food on his list, and again it is Pacific oysters.[64] I would recommend moving up just one notch in his list and boosting your immune system with oyster mushrooms.

The Great Debate

I have provided you with my responses to the differing nutritional philosophies of Drs. Lufkin, Means, Hyman, and Li. It is time now to address the "sticky wicket" that I alluded to earlier: If we all agree, along with a growing body of health experts and even politicians, that nutrition should be taught in medical school, but we have differing nutritional ideologies, exactly whose ideas of nutrition should be taught?

First, let's keep in mind that there are vital parts of a nutritional curriculum that should not be contentious: the nutritional constituents of foods, for example. The nutritional needs of bodily organs can usually be agreed upon as well; there's no dispute, for example, that the thyroid requires iodine. The debate truly begins when we address how best to construct a diet that optimizes human health and longevity.

Of course, scientific truth is not determined by debate. It is determined by data. The final criterion as to healthiness of a diet would be to observe an obvious benefit in lifespan, and more importantly, health span. That is, a difference in the years of high-functioning, relatively disease-free life, in a group following one dietary style compared with another. The definitive study to determine that would be to follow a significant number (at least 2,500 or more) of omnivores of different stripes (those on keto, Paleo, and Mediterranean diets, for example) and an equal number of practitioners of a WPF diet over the course of their lives to learn the cause of the illnesses they acquire and their actual causes of death.

During this study, ideally of lifetime length, researchers would have to keep track of what each participant was actually eating, since wildly differing patterns within the "omnivore" or "plant-exclusive" categories could be associated with various disease causations or preventions. Ideally, the subjects would need to remain faithful to their diets for their lifetimes—a daunting challenge to the study design, to say the least. Other lifestyle factors—such as exercise, sleep, stress, work satisfaction, relationship status, and connection to a community—would also need to be documented and factored into the analysis. Theoretically, this magnificent study would yield the reliable answers we seek regarding the "omnivore vs. whole plant food" outcomes.

And, of course, such a study will never be done. It would require scores of researchers following thousands of people over decades at a cost of untold millions of dollars. Who is going to fund such a study? Big Broccoli? No one will make mega dollars by telling the public to eat more vegetables, and, again, such a study seems almost impossibly difficult to undertake.

Since we are lacking the definitive evidence that would be provided by this longitudinal study, the best that we can do is to draw conclusions from publicly available morbidity and mortality statistics, and from various dietary recall studies like the EPIC-Oxford and Adventist Health studies. In these studies, participants are sent questionnaires every year in hopes of recalling accurately what they have been eating in the past twelve months. (I can't recall what I had for lunch yesterday.)

In many such studies, the number of vegans is so small that they are lumped in with the vegetarian subjects and, therefore, cannot be accurately characterized regarding health outcomes and lifespans. This is certainly the case in "Mortality in British Vegetarians: Results from the European Prospective Investigation into Cancer and Nutrition (EPIC-Oxford)." That study stated in the statistical analysis sections that "the vegans are included with the vegetarians because there were too few deaths among the vegans to report separately."[65] Moreover, vegans are certainly not always practicing a WPF diet, so "junk food vegans" would be skewing the data and perhaps rendering it almost meaningless.

Consequently, the ammunition that each side hurls at the other in the "dueling studies" contests is generally of very poor quality and quite inadequate to settle the argument one way or another. That may be good for podcasts, but it does little for science. We must be open to trying other methods to reach consensus.

Here's my suggestion: The medical community should address the matter in a manner analogous to the way the courts address legal arguments. One side presents a brief; the other side responds to the brief with its counterarguments; then the first side answers the counterarguments; and so forth. Formal debates follow a similar methodology. Medical schools could thereby utilize a nutritional curriculum that, in addressing the subject of the optimal human diet, would read like the competing briefs of a court case. This would allow the students to make up their own minds as they follow the arguments along. Suddenly, nutrition would be transformed from an obscure subject that medical schools effectively shun into the vibrant center of a medical education, and students would be energized to join the debate. I fervently wish that had been the case when I was in medical school.

On the plant-exclusive side of the argument, I foresee no difficulty in forging an argument that explains all the reasons by which we know that human beings are natural herbivores, and all the ways in which a WPF diet can prevent and reverse the metabolic disorders that are costing our country the bulk of the $5 trillion that we spend on healthcare in order to achieve the lowest life expectancy of peer nations and forty-ninth place in the world.[66, 67] I'm confident that the Plantrician Project, the American College of Lifestyle Medicine, and the Physicians Committee for Responsible Medicine, perhaps along with other leading lights of our movement, would gladly cooperate in creating such a document.

The other side, advocating animal foods as part, or most, or all of the human diet, will be trickier to corral. The keto diet allows dairy but little or no fruit. The Paleo diet does not allow dairy but embraces fruit, and it promotes a diet that is considerably less fatty than the keto diet (though fattier than the WPF diet). The carnivore diet, if it deserves to be taken seriously, allows no plant foods at all, believe it or not. So perhaps the animal-food-friendly side will have to file multiple "briefs" to accommodate all of its competing sects. Perhaps a committee of medical school deans can decide which "sects" deserve representation, and/or a method could be implemented to allow something resembling "*amicus curae*" briefs to be filed by those who don't feel their views have been adequately represented.

Each side should be allowed to flag certain of their own arguments as a way of demanding that those specific arguments be responded to by the opposition. Let me give you an example of the kind of argument that the WPF side might make, and why a response must be insisted upon.

In 1913, a Russian scientist named Nikolay Nikolayevich Anichkov, working at a lab in St. Petersburg, conducted a powerfully important experiment. He fed cholesterol from egg yolks to some poor, unsuspecting rabbits. The rabbits developed atherosclerotic plaque and lesions.

It was subsequently proven that cholesterol fed to omnivores and carnivores, such as dogs and cats, does not cause atherosclerosis to develop.

Atherosclerosis, therefore, is a disease that develops only in herbivores.

Atherosclerosis develops, of course, in humans, manifesting as heart disease and related maladies. In fact, humans are the only mammals that suffer (when leading their natural lives, free of confinement)[68] from atherosclerosis, which could be defined as an arterial disease that develops when an herbivore is fed a steady diet of animal foods. And—*what do you know!*—we happen to be the only mammal that fits that definition.

Therefore, humans are herbivores.

That is an argument to which the other side must respond. They have to explain logically how it has come to be that only humans, of all mammals living free lives and eating their instinctive diets, develop atherosclerosis, and they have to explain why we shouldn't deduce from Anichkov's work that we are natural herbivores. I've yet to hear a compelling response, although I'll note that Dr. Lufkin takes a feeble stab at it in *Lies I Taught in Medical School,* in which he writes:

> Anichkov's work has since been recognized as one of medicine's ten greatest discoveries. Another author called it one of "cardiology's ten greatest discoveries of the twentieth century."
>
> The accolades are impressive, except that the work is based on an error. These authors overlooked the fact that rabbits are herbivores (or plant eaters), for which cholesterol was a foreign material in their diets . . . When researchers attempted to replicate the experiment on omnivores such as dogs (and humans) who had cholesterol as part of their normal diets, the results were mixed . . .[69]

Excuse me? Does Dr. Lufkin seriously believe that Anichkov, or the authors who praised his work, did not realize that rabbits were herbivores? The fact that atherosclerosis could be generated in this way in the herbivorous rabbits (but not in the omnivorous dogs) is the *whole point*, not an "error."

Can the other side come up with a better, more logical response than Dr. Lufkin's? I'm champing at the bit to find out.

The WPF side must demand an answer, too, to the case we make that stems from an analysis of comparative anatomy. For decades, our side has pointed to the innumerable ways in which a comparison of the anatomy of mammalian herbivores, mammalian omnivores, and mammalian carnivores leads to the inescapable conclusion that humans are herbivores. I alluded to this in chapter 2, but there are far more anatomical examples than I mentioned. Carnivores have short gastrointestinal tracts to allow them to relatively quickly expel the animal food they kill, and they are able to secrete enough hydrochloric acid to keep their gastric acidity in the range of 1–2, to quell the bacteria in flesh foods.[70] Humans, like other herbivores, have long intestinal tracts and much milder stomach acidity.

Like other herbivores, we do not have the wide oral gape of carnivores, or the dentition of carnivores, or the hinged jaw motion of carnivores. We do not possess claws. We do not have the short gestation period of carnivores, which allows for hunting. Herbivores can see color, so that we can detect tasty fruit, for example; carnivores and omnivores have heightened visual ability to detect movement (important when you are stalking prey) but not color.

There are many more ways in which humans align with all mammalian herbivores rather than with carnivores and omnivores. If you search online for "Dr. Milton Mills: Are We Designed to Eat Meat?" you will find an excellent lecture by Dr. Mills on the subject.[71] I would dearly love, for the first time in human history, to see Dr. Mills's arguments answered by the other side. It will, in any case, be enlightening to watch them try.

With each side of the nutritional divide presenting arguments and inviting responses, not only would the curriculum on nutrition in medical school be science based, but there would also be a rigorous and scientific approach to its presentation based on the sciences of comparative anatomy, evolutionary biology, molecular biology, molecular biochemistry, genetics, epidemiology, and more.

We have seen that a growing consensus exists in the medical community that good metabolism presents the key to health. A growing consensus exists, too, that nutrition must be taught, and emphasized, in medical school. Nonetheless, the nutrition wars continue unabated, providing at the very least an excuse for the deans of medical schools not to address these emerging consensuses. That is why I propose that we teach nutrition in medical school in a way that gives all sides ample opportunity to present their case, in a curriculum that aligns with the rules of debate as well as the methods of science. Let the better arguments carry the day, while we truly augment the education of future doctors by trusting and engaging their powers of critical thinking, rather than just rote memorization.

What Teaching Nutrition Looks Like

All that being said, one final argument needs to be addressed. In suggesting to medical school deans that nutrition should be taught in medical school, their response has frequently been: "The curriculum for these students is already jam-packed with courses. Which ones do you want us to omit to make room for your nutrition courses? Anatomy? Physiology? There just isn't any room for nutrition courses . . ."

In fact, there is no need to drop any course at all—just incorporate applied nutrition into all four years of medical school studies. That is, in the first year, when anatomy, physiology, and biochemistry are taught, the structure and function of the digestive system as it turns food into energy should be highlighted in each subject. When pharmacology is taught, a rigorous look at how food and, say, obesity affect the pharmacokinetics of drugs should be essential. Certainly, in pathology, the contribution of the patient's diet to most of the diseases that are studied should be incorporated into the etiology of the illnesses.

When the student moves into the clinical rotations in the third and fourth years, each specialty should have clinics and lectures highlighting the role of diet in each of the medical conditions seen. On the obstetrics rotation, it should be taught that a woman's diet is a direct determinant of whether she develops gestational diabetes and whether her baby will be overnourished and macrosomic (too large for the birth canal), necessitating a caesarean section. In pediatrics, understanding the child's diet will be central to helping them avoid or overcome many chronic diseases, from asthma to type 2 diabetes to incipient coronary artery disease—which, by the way, has tragically become a pediatric disease, given the Standard American Diet eaten by children on a daily basis. It should become obvious on the rotations through surgery and internal medicine that diet plays a key role in creating the diseases for which the patient seeks treatment.

In this way, nutrition would be woven into every course of study throughout the medical school years, with the result of the school graduating a physician truly capable of understanding—and helping the patient to reverse—most of the diseases they will be seeing in their career.

If you would like to help create a revolutionary change in the teaching of medicine, please go to MovingMedForward.org and sign up for our newsletter, *The Forward Report.* We'll keep you informed about actions you can take. But certainly, the most important thing everyone can do is to eat a WPF diet, achieve admirable health, and serve as a beacon to friends and family.

Chapter Seven

A DAY AT THE DISEASE REVERSAL CLINIC

A "disease reversal clinic" is a fictional entity at the moment. But let us hope it will soon become a standard fixture in medical centers everywhere. And in truth, every doctor's office and clinic can and should be a "disease reversal clinic." So, in the following pages, I want to envision for my fellow physicians and allied health professionals a way to realize the dreams of physicians through the ages—to truly banish disease from the body and life of their patients. And for anyone dissatisfied with their own healthcare, consider this an aspirational example of what could be, and perhaps an inspiration for starting an important conversation with your own physician.

These are the words I wish my chief resident would have said to me when I was starting my rotation on outpatient medicine. It would have changed the course of my career.

Welcome to the DRC

Hello, new colleagues. Let me introduce you to a clinic experience that may well alter your understanding of your role as physician, and demonstrate how you can work with your patients to help them improve their own health.

This is not your standard internal medicine ward or cardiology service where we play musical chairs with medications and chase numbers on lab reports. Here, at the disease reversal clinic, the DRC, we do something radical: We treat the cause of disease.

The patients you'll see in this clinic are not unique cases; they are the norm in modern medicine increasingly around the globe, commonly suffering with obesity, hypertension, type 2 diabetes, atherosclerosis, and a host of inflammatory and autoimmune disorders. But what sets this clinic apart is that we don't merely manage these conditions—we reverse them. And we do it without the ever-expanding polypharmacy regimen that traditional medicine relies upon. Instead, our primary tools are positive lifestyle practices and a diet composed predominantly of whole plant foods.

The SAD Story

Before we go out and see our patients, let's take a few minutes to consider the science behind why this approach works so effectively to routinely accomplish what, until recently, was considered impossible: the reversal of chronic disease.

As I suspect you already know, the main driving cause of most of the illnesses people bring to you in the DRC is the Standard American Diet, SAD. A tailor-made recipe for chronic disease, the SAD is calorically dense but nutritionally bankrupt, loaded with processed foods, animal fats and proteins, refined sugars and oils, and excessive sodium.

So, let's briefly analyze the conditions caused when this toxic fuel mix pours through the tissues after every fast-food and restaurant meal, day after day, year after year, unleashing most of the chronic diseases you are going to spend your medical careers treating.

Obesity

As the abundant saturated fats in the SAD repeatedly pour through the abdominal fat stores, they are taken up by the adipocytes (fat cells) resident there. The SAD excels only in this one way—as a diabolically effective obesogenic diet: high in calorie-dense foods, hyperpalatable on the tongue, low in fiber, and virtually absent of satiety-inducing whole plant foods. This combination of hyperpalatable, ultra-processed foods and chronic caloric excess dysregulates the balance between leptin and ghrelin, the hormones governing hunger and satiety. This imbalance contributes to overeating and the resulting metabolic dysfunction. The results are evident in the expanding waistlines we see all around us, increasingly normalized by the media and advertisers.

Atherosclerosis and Cardiovascular Disease

Frequently eating SAD foods is a direct assault on the vascular system. Saturated fats from animal products elevate atherogenic LDL cholesterol and promote endothelial dysfunction and arterial plaque formation. Meanwhile, the lack of antioxidant-rich plant foods allows oxidative stress and inflammation in the artery walls to further drive atherosclerosis.[1] The saturated fats, along with refined carbohydrates and sugars, also contribute to insulin resistance with resulting hyperglycemia, which further accelerates cardiovascular damage.

Hypertension

Processed foods, such as prepared meats, cheeses, chips, and most fast foods, are laden with refined oils and salt and are deficient in potassium. When they are eaten, the sudden salt load has two adverse effects upon the vascular system: one, the sodium atoms from the salt enter the artery wall, pulling water molecules in along with them, producing a micro-edema within the blood vessel wall, stiffening it, and making it less able to relax between heartbeats; two, in order to dilute the salt load in the blood, the kidneys retain water they would otherwise excrete in the urine, thus increasing the total volume of blood to be pumped by the heart. These problems are exacerbated by the saturated fats and vegetable oils that can promote endothelial dysfunction, further reducing nitric oxide availability, leading to chronic vasoconstriction. The heart, now forced to pump a larger volume of blood through miles of stiffened, contracted arteries, must do so at a higher pressure. After years of pumping against this increased vascular resistance, the ventricular walls thicken, and the ventricular myocytes become attenuated and infiltrated with fibrous tissue; eventually, congestive heart failure can result.

Type 2 Diabetes

The SAD fuels insulin resistance through excessive saturated fat intake, which penetrates into liver and muscle cells and impairs insulin receptor function. The resulting hyperinsulinemia (excess insulin in the blood) eventually leads to beta-cell exhaustion and, ultimately, full-blown type 2 diabetes.[2]

Autoimmune and Inflammatory Diseases

A diet high in processed meats, dairy, refined oils, and excessive sodium triggers chronic inflammation through numerous mechanisms, including absorption of pro-inflammatory compounds like Neu5Gc, endotoxin, and arachidonic acid. The gut microbiota, shaped largely by the patient's diet, also plays a pivotal role in immune function. A diet heavy with meat and eggs fosters the growth of microbes that can inflame the gut wall, resulting in increased gut permeability. These mechanisms can open the door to such autoimmune pathologies as lupus and inflammatory bowel disease.[3]

Disease Reversal

How do we help our patient's body reverse these disease processes?

The good news, as I suspect you know since you're working here in the DRC, is that all of the above serious chronic diseases can often be arrested, and sometimes even reversed, through dietary and positive lifestyle practices. Let me be clear that I am not claiming that a whole plant food diet is a panacea that will magically stop all lethal diseases in their tracks and restore youthful health and function. A body shot through with metastatic cancer or a brain riddled with Alzheimer's plaques may be beyond disease reversal, though a WPF diet can, through its anti-inflammatory properties, create improvements in a number of symptoms, even in these advanced cases. But, like all therapies, the effects of a WPF-based program will depend upon how enthusiastically it is embraced and instituted by the patient.

What is the source of the disease-reversing powers of the WPF diet? A food stream composed mostly of whole plant foods is naturally rich in fiber, antioxidants, and anti-inflammatory compounds, and all of those components will work in concert to restore metabolic health.

Let's suppose that your patient has made a complete transition away from all animal products, and they have fully adopted a WPF diet. The most important change their body experiences is that the previous, every-four-hour deluge of food-based nutritional saboteurs from meat, dairy, and processed foods (the "Toxic Red Tide") stops. Finally, they achieve respite from the repeated toxic floods from the SAD meals. Now there is time, utilizing the phytonutrients supplied by the whole plant foods, for healing to be promoted on the cellular level in every tissue. Let's consider even a few of the positive clinical changes that predictably occur as the components of the whole plant food stream now flood your patient's body with every meal.

Achieving Healthy Weight Loss

Because Mother Nature cleverly makes fruits and vegetables, legumes, and grains mostly out of fiber and water, not surprisingly, a whole plant food diet is mostly made of fiber and water. Consequently, it is a food stream naturally lower in calorie density. Yet, because it is high in fiber, it leads to greater satiety more quickly and, over time, reduced overall caloric intake. Fiber also slows gastric emptying and modulates appetite hormones, further facilitating sustainable weight loss without a feeling of deprivation.[4] As a result of all the foregoing mechanisms, people who adopt the whole plant food diet predictably shed excess body fat. Within twelve to twenty-four months, they usually arrive at, and maintain, their ideal body weight. That makes this style of eating joyous and guilt free: no calorie counting, no "carb counting"; if your patient goes back for a third bowl of vegetable soup, who cares? A broth-based vegetable soup will consist mostly of fiber and water, which pass through your patient's body without adding to their fat stores, while the phytonutrients in the vegetables nourish the body's cells.

Healing the Vascular Tree

Fortunately, the artery endothelium is capable of remarkable self-repair. Remember, the bone marrow constantly releases showers of stem cells that can "reupholster" the artery linings, like new paving stones placed during a road repair. Because the stem cells operate under the influence of chemical messengers released by the injured surface of the artery lining, they transform themselves into healthy endothelial cells. Over time, the smooth, nitric oxide–rich lining is restored, along with the elastic properties of the artery wall.

The artery repair process is further bolstered by the nitric oxide–boosting foods, especially leafy greens and beets, in the whole plant food diet that you will be recommending to your patient. Also working in your patient's favor are the fiber and phytochemicals that tend to lower LDL cholesterol and help reduce arterial plaque. Like a sandbar dissolving in the strong, steady flow of a river's current, atherosclerotic plaques in the artery walls really can melt away under the daily flow of phytonutrient-rich, inflammation-quenching antioxidants inherent in the whole plant food diet.[5]

Lowering Blood Pressure Naturally

Potassium-rich plant foods (sweet potatoes, legumes, and bananas are good examples) and magnesium-rich leafy greens counteract sodium-induced hypertension. Additionally, the whole plant food diet, with its abundant soups, stews, salads, cooked grains, steamed vegetables, and fruits, is a high-water-content food stream. By adding more water to the bloodstream, it reduces blood viscosity.[6] This allows the heart to propel the more free-flowing blood along at a lower pressure. This mechanism alone can help lower blood pressure without medication.[7]

Restoring Insulin Sensitivity

By sharply reducing the dietary saturated fats that inhibit insulin receptors in the muscles and liver, and replacing them with whole carbohydrates, a whole plant food diet allows the insulin receptors on the muscle and liver cells to regain normal function, thus reversing insulin resistance. In many, if not most, cases, assuming normal insulin production by the pancreas, over time, type 2 diabetes can resolve completely. In some cases, patients can come off insulin injections within weeks by following a controlled tapering regimen. Physicians will need to learn the essential craft of "de-prescribing" insulin as well as other potent hypoglycemic medications.

Guidance for tapering off insulin and other hypoglycemic agents can be found at Deprescribing.org, as well as in medical literature.

Calming the Immune System and Quelling Inflammation

How does a fiber-rich diet promote a healthy gut microbiome? A whole plant food stream, especially rich in resistant starches in legumes, cooked potatoes, and pastas, fosters the replacement of more pro-inflammatory microbes from the phyla *Bacteroidetes* with those of the *Prevotella* family. The byproducts that the *Prevotella* microbes produce reduce gut permeability as well as the amount of endotoxin that leaks into the bloodstream and lymphatic flow, thus minimizing systemic inflammation. It has become a common experience among autoimmune patients to experience significant symptom relief—or even complete remission of their syndrome—by adopting a plant-predominant diet. Many patients have found dramatic improvement in their lupus and other autoimmune and inflammatory conditions by utilizing the protocols in *Goodbye Autoimmune Disease* by Dr. Brooke Goldner, a physician who put her own severe lupus into remission with a regimen of a largely raw, WPF diet and green smoothies.

Practicing Lifestyle Medicine

I hope that, by now, you understand that this plant-predominant food stream can effectively reverse chronic disease in many, if not most of your patients, and it should be the underpinning of any health-restoring treatment you recommend. Fortunately, there are not separate, distinct WPF diets for diabetes reversal, atherosclerosis reversal, and hypertension reversal. Here, for the most part, one size really does fit all, although of course individualization for each person's health condition and food preferences must still be taken into account and the diet tweaked regarding its contents of fat, sodium, and other components. Consultation and guidance from a plant-aware registered dietitian can be invaluable.

Remember, the WPF diet derives its disease-reversing power from the daily surges of antioxidant-rich nutrients that flood through the body's cells with every vegetable-laden salad, soup, and serving of dark leafy greens. Unlike the animal-based Toxic Red Tide that visits repeated cellular injury upon the organs with every burger and bratwurst, the plant-plentiful dishes of the WPF diet bathe the cells, meal after meal, week after week, with a free-flowing, nutrient-rich stream, delivering healing micronutrients that quench free radicals, soothe inflamed tissues, and promote healing on the cellular level throughout the body. This sets the stage for the dramatic remissions so often seen in the disease reversal clinic.

Now that you understand something about the powerful tools and mechanisms you have at your disposal to reverse disease in your patients, let's talk about what you'll actually do in the DRC—and in your own practice if that is where you are headed. Nothing should surprise you here:

1. Take a proper medical history.
2. Perform a physical examination appropriate to your setting (in-person appointment vs. telemedicine session).
3. Evaluate lab results and any imaging findings.
4. Arrive at a diagnosis.
5. Institute a treatment plan based upon the principles of lifestyle medicine.

Let's consider what this looks like in the real world.

Patient Intake and Medical History

Patients should have filled out a questionnaire describing their current dietary and lifestyle practices. Be thoroughly familiar with this before you first see your patient. Keys to the cause and eventual treatment of their conditions often lie in the responses found on the food and lifestyle questionnaire.

When the patient is in front of you, either in person or via telemedicine, make a human connection. Let them feel your concern, both as a physician and as a fellow human being, acknowledging that we all simply do the best we can. Let them know that they will never feel judgment or a "finger-wag" from you. Make it clear that you are unconditionally on their side as they progress towards better health. Beyond their medical and nutritional history, explore the realities of their family life, their work, their sources of stress, and their ways of coping with it. Try to get a sense of their overall happiness with their life and career.

What role does food play in their life? Always inquire about who does the shopping and cooking in their house, what their favorite foods are, and what food cravings they contend with. Be sure to ask what they believe constitutes a healthy diet.

Red Flags

As you assess your new patient, be on the lookout for signs of acute medical decompensation from progressive congestive heart failure or chronic kidney disease (CKD) that may lie under the surface. As the medical adage reminds us, "All that wheezes is not asthma, and all fatigue is not from lack of sleep." Though the context of the appointment is "lifestyle medicine," the specter of serious medical diseases is ever present. Specifically inquire about chest pain, shortness of breath, arrhythmias, or any other concerning symptoms. Be especially vigilant for signs of significant systemic changes, such as a sudden increase in fatigue, fevers, or pain. Take a thorough travel history and always review all medications being taken. Keep in mind that "polypharmacy" is a common cause of fatigue, nausea, unsteadiness, and many other symptoms.

As far as practical, conduct a physical examination. If the person is physically present, pay close attention to the examination of the heart, lungs, thyroid, and liver. If it is a telemedicine consultation, assess their facial symmetry, range of motion of joints, edema of ankles, coloration of skin, and ease of breathing. It is usually wise to arrange for home blood pressure monitoring and for the patient to send the recorded readings to your office on a monthly basis. Recognizing the sensitivity many patients have around their weight, dispassionately record the patient's weight at each visit and, when appropriate, ask the person how they are feeling about their weight. As their weight is recorded, it is often helpful to ask the person what they believe caused any change in their weight, whether it went up or down.

Key Questions

Don't neglect the other pillars of a healthy lifestyle. At your first visit with the patient—and at each follow-up visit—be sure to inquire about the other aspects of the patient's life that contribute to optimal health.

1. Physical activity: Are they at least getting outside for a thirty-minute walk each day? Are they doing anything to maintain their flexibility and muscle strength? Ask about the realities in their life and be ready with simple suggestions to help them move more.
2. Restorative sleep: Are they getting seven or eight hours of restful sleep each night?
3. Stress management: Ask about their levels and sources of stress. Make what useful suggestions you can for managing it, but often, just your listening to their narration of their stressful situation can be therapeutic for them.
4. Social connection: Ask about what social support network exists for them. Are they close with family, friends, workmates, or teammates? If they are bereft of social support, make

recommendations about local and online resources that are available to them.

5. Avoidance of risky substances: Ask about their use of cigarettes, alcohol, drugs, and other injurious agents and discuss with them ways to discontinue their use.
6. The natural world: Ask if they spend any time out in nature as an additional pillar to bring serenity and balance into their lives.

Your spending time briefly discussing these six aspects of their daily life can prove as important as your guidance regarding their food choices. All of these factors play their part in the tasks at hand for the concerned physician: disease prevention and disease reversal.

To find out what your patient has really been eating, requesting that they bring in a three-day food diary, which you and the patient will both review during the visit, can prove quite revelatory for both doctor and patient.

If indicated, order and evaluate appropriate laboratory tests.

Lab Tests

If laboratory tests have already been performed, review them to help complete the diagnostic picture. This is a good time to evaluate any data from the patient's continuous glucose monitor (CGM) or other wearable devices to gain a better understanding of the person's physiology. If further lab tests or imaging are required, make a note to order them. But as always: "If it's not going to change your treatment, don't order the tests."

Here are some guidelines for the laboratory tests and their recommended intervals as you follow your patient over the months and years:

1. Fasting glucose or hemoglobin HgbA1c. The HgbA1c provides a picture of the average blood sugar control over the past two to three months.

2. Lipid profile. This panel should include: LDL, HDL, total cholesterol, ApoB number, LP(a), and triglycerides. To check for arterial plaque–associated inflammation, also measure: high sensitivity C-reactive protein (HS-CRP) and myeloperoxidase (MPO).
3. Liver function tests. Nonalcoholic fatty liver disease (NAFLD) is common in patients with metabolic syndrome, obesity, and insulin resistance. Testing bilirubin, albumin, AST, ALT, GGT, and alkaline phosphatase can help assess liver health and is generally done annually, unless more frequent monitoring is needed.
4. Renal function tests. Test serum creatinine and eGFR (estimated glomerular filtration rate) along with a urinalysis annually.
5. Insulin levels and insulin resistance. Tests like fasting insulin and calculations for insulin resistance (e.g., HOMA-IR) can be useful, especially in the baseline evaluation. Measure insulin resistance if HgbA1c readings stay elevated. Also, a falling level of insulin resistance will cheer both the doctor and the patient as they see their healthy-lifestyle strategies paying off.
6. Complete blood count (CBC). This will check for anemia and infection.
7. B-type natriuretic peptide (BNP). If congestive heart failure is suspected, this test is valuable.
8. Electrocardiogram. This should be ordered if the patient is suffering chest pain or arrhythmia. Keep in mind that a high percentage of EKGs will read "abnormal," and so a mere "abnormal" reading is not necessarily a cause for alarm. But if there is any serious clinical concern, do not hesitate to refer the patient to a cardiologist or to the ER.

Diagnosis

By this time, you should have a good idea of the state of the patient's health. In modern America, expect to consistently encounter obesity, atherosclerotic vascular disease, type 2 diabetes, fatty liver disease, hypertension, and various manifestations of inflammatory and/or autoimmune diseases. You will have some good news to deliver to the patient, who will find it motivating to learn that they have the power to arrest and reverse these maladies with proper diet and lifestyle practices.

After considering the information gathered through the medical history, physical exam, and laboratory results, a diagnosis will take form in your mind. Always remember that the body is a dynamic, constantly changing system, so hold each diagnostic possibility lightly and with humility, ready to abandon it without hesitation when a more likely mechanism or explanation presents itself. You have no obligation except to the truth and to the care of your patient.

As always in medicine, beware of diagnoses ossifying in your mind: "This patient has xyz disease and what we are seeing is because xyz disease does that." Although that may well prove correct, looking at only the primary diagnosis may lead us to miss new situations developing. Always do a quick head-to-toe exam when possible and make sure that everything you are seeing clinically is explained by the diagnoses attached to the patient. If something doesn't fit, then further investigation is indicated.

Develop a Treatment Program

With the diagnosis made, it is time to marshal the forces of healing—both on the part of the doctor and the patient. Stress to the patient that they must be a full partner in their own healing. Knowledge alone won't reverse disease—behavioral change will.

Do not be shy in using prescription medications if they are temporarily necessary to control currently problematic symptoms, such as hypertension or hyperglycemia. But be sure to share with your patient that the prescriptions you are issuing are being given with the intent of only being a temporary bridge to keep them safe while they get themselves healthier with a WPF diet and positive lifestyle changes.

When the patient hears that your prescription is not "lifetime medication," they usually feel a sense of relief along with empowerment over their own health future and motivation to work with you to make progress.

Explain the patient's health condition to them clearly, especially the diet-disease link. Use visual aids to ensure that the person understands the nature of their health challenge. Let the patient know you will be their ally throughout their medical journey and will guide them through treatments and referrals, if such are required. Most of all, give them encouragement.

Tell your patients the truth, even when it's uncomfortable. Patients aren't fragile. Be direct, while being compassionate and solution focused. Your patients will appreciate such insight as:

"Your high blood pressure isn't from a lack of medication—it's from what's on your plate."

"Your diabetes isn't genetic—it's from years of insulin resistance caused by eating fatty foods."

"Your child isn't 'big for their age'—they're on track for metabolic disease before high school."

Let them know that medications they are on may be maintained or changed, but that together you will be striving towards the ultimate goal of the patient achieving a level of health such that they do not need the medications at all. (Be prepared to learn the techniques of "deprescribing" mentioned previously.)

Have a thorough and honest discussion with your patient about making what may well need to be dramatic changes in their dietary habits. Ask them how ready they are to make such healthy changes in their food choices, and what they believe are their biggest barriers to successfully doing so.

Let them know that theirs is not an "all or nothing" situation. Creating long-term health is a marathon, not a sprint. Consistent, incremental diet and lifestyle changes can make for true and sustainable progress. Celebrate every small victory with them. At the same time, make sure they understand that they cannot expect dramatic health improvements with only minor tweaks to a profoundly unhealthy diet.

Provide them with handouts, recipes, and other support materials.

Let them know you want to see them back in three to four weeks for follow-up and that you are always available to them for support. Then refer them to a registered dietitian, and ask your patient to connect with the RD as soon as possible to develop their food program.

Working with Plant-Aware Registered Dietitians

A team approach is essential for success in lifestyle medicine. Find your registered dietitian colleagues through online searches for "plant-based registered dietitians" or through organizations like the Plantrician Project, the American College of Lifestyle Medicine, and the Physicians Committee for Responsible Medicine. These RDs are trained professionals who will do the required initial nutritional counseling for you, and they are especially valuable for patients with complex medical situations, such as those with diabetes, inflammatory bowel disease, fatty liver disease, and advanced atherosclerosis. Since diet counseling works well through telemedicine, the dietitian does not even have to be in the same city as you—but of course must have a valid license in the patient's state.

You are encouraged to establish a professional referral arrangement with one or more of these plant-aware dietitians and schedule times to receive their feedback and suggestions about the patients you have referred.

More and more health insurers will cover the cost of an RD consultation, so be sure to check in with the patient and the RD to verify that the service is covered. However, given that the RD can provide invaluable nutritional guidance in just a visit or two, even paying out of pocket is usually well worth the cost.

Working with Food Coaches

With the physician focused on promoting medical improvements, and the registered dietitian tracking nutrient intakes and food-drug interactions, it is likely that neither of these two professionals has time to field the individual patient's queries about handling the practical and psychological challenges involved in adopting a diet. Especially a diet that not only may be utterly new to the patient but also places them squarely—at least for now—in the dietary minority.

Food coaches are an optional asset to the treatment plan, but they can be invaluable. The role of the food coach is to make sure the dietary protocols prescribed by the doctor and dietitian are actually followed—and to help the patient/client overcome the real-world obstacles that inevitably arise. The food coach is the motivational guide who helps their client succeed, not someone who alters the treatment plan or suggests supplements to take. Your patient will be more likely to stay on their game if they know that, in their weekly call with the food coach, they will be asked:

1. How did their previous week go, foodwise?
2. What worked and what didn't?
3. What obstacles did they encounter that prevented healthy eating in a given situation?
4. If their weight changed, up or down, what do they think accounted for that change?
5. What do they need to become happier and more confident and effective in their food choices?

To my knowledge, there are no national or state standards or certifications for food coaches, but often these coaches have obtained certifications from one of the organizations listed in this book's resources section (see p. 211). Usually, the services of the food coach are needed only for a few weeks or months. But those who use the service generally feel it is money well spent.

With the food coach providing frequent, personalized support for the patient, and communicating regularly with the RD and MD/DO, the health professionals may only need to see the patient every few months until they are stable.

Establishing Trust with a Reluctant Patient

For those white-knuckled patients who tremble at the thought of changing their current diet and lifestyle choices, you can assure them that perfection isn't necessary. If 80 percent of their diet shifts to whole plant foods, their health will drastically transform for the better. This is known as the "80/20 strategy." Let them know that they can still enjoy occasional indulgences without guilt—but encourage them to hold the food debauches to a minimum, as in once or twice a week, at the most.

Of course, make it clear to them that there will be added benefit as their diet continues to become more plant exclusive. I suggest the 80/20 strategy only as an initial soft-landing plan for the average, reluctant-to-change omnivore, not as a permanent lifestyle. At each visit, I inquire if the patient's feeling better overall and, if they are (a usual occurrence), I have them share how they feel about it, discussing what change or action accounted for their progress—and then, I celebrate their victory with them.

The best way to prove that plant-based food isn't a sacrifice is to let people taste it. Recommend sumptuous, satisfying alternatives to animal foods, like a filling lentil chili instead of beef chili or a flavorful portobello burger instead of a beef patty. Some of my lifestyle medicine colleagues even use their office waiting area after hours as a mini teaching kitchen for their patients on the plant-based journey. They set up tables and bring in blenders, hot plates, and Instant Pots, to show people how to prepare smoothies, salad dressings, grains, and soups—and let them taste each one. A taste is worth a thousand words! And these real-time demonstrations are often the convincer in helping people move to healthier eating. When you hear a taste-testing patient say: "Wow. If that is plant-based food, I could definitely eat that!" then you know real progress is being made. Be ready to supply recipes and links to plant-based food websites.

For the skeptic, let the results do the talking. A powerful motivator is to start tracking your patient's lab markers. Watching with the patient as their levels of cholesterol, blood sugar, and blood pressure improve over the weeks provides inspiration. Likewise, your lowering—and eventually, discontinuing—their medication will be an added, joyful validation of their progress.

Encourage their family or supporters to join in by enjoying the same food and helping with the shopping and meal preparation. When loved ones are on board, transitions become much easier and more enjoyable.

By meeting patients where they are and helping them make gradual, sustainable changes, you'll not only improve their health—you'll also transform their lives.

Chapter Eight

IT JUST SO HAPPENS

I noted in chapter 6 that the author Gary Taubes, who favors the (usually meat-based) ketogenic diet, concedes that a vegan diet leaves a far lighter environmental footprint. From his point of view, I suppose, *it just so happens* that the animal-food-based diet he has spent decades advocating turns out to be—*bad luck!*—an unmitigated disaster for our environment and our climate, not to mention being very unfortunate for the animals involved.

It just so happens, as well, that a plant-based diet can feed the world far more efficiently than an animal-based diet, as farmers can grow upwards of 4,000 percent more plant food than meat per acre.[1] All the grain currently cycled through animals could be used to feed humans directly, leading to far greater efficiency and dramatically less hunger. Since it would require so much less land to feed humans a plant-based diet, the saved land, formerly grazed by animals (in the United States, that would be about half our continental land mass), could be rewilded, allowing so many more trees and so much more vegetation to grow that *it just so happens* that enough carbon dioxide could be sequestered to actually reverse climate change,[2] which is currently advancing on a seemingly unstoppable path that presents an existential threat to civilization.

One can also adopt the view that it's an unlucky coincidence—in other words, *it just so happens*—that most pandemics have their origin in animal agriculture. Pandemics often begin because "food animals" have been crowded together in unnatural conditions and have been put in close contact with human beings. At this writing, researchers, epidemiologists, and public health officials struggle to contain the H5N1 bird flu. There have now been over sixty human cases, and one human death, in the United States from this avian flu (with hundreds of human deaths worldwide), while bird deaths are currently estimated at around three hundred million. As *The Guardian* points out, "The origins of all highly pathogenic avian influenzas—the ones that cause severe disease and death—have been tracked back to poultry farms."[3] Sea lions, seals, cats, dogs, cows, tigers, and other animals have also been victims of the outbreak.

Of course, we humans possess, in our arsenal, a potent weapon against nonviral pandemics, as well as against other bacterial diseases: antibiotics. They can also be useful during viral pandemics, in that bacterial infections can appear in conjunction with viral outbreaks. Moreover, there is reason for concern that future pandemics may prove to be bacterial, rather than viral, in nature.[4] But we now face the dilemma that our antibiotics may fail us, since the profligate use of antibiotics has led to antibiotic resistance in pathogens. And *it just so happens* that by far the most profligate use of antibiotics stems from animal agriculture, where antibiotics are used both to help fatten animals and to help prevent disease when "food animals" are crowded together obscenely.

Of course, a strong natural immune system remains our most potent weapon against all forms of disease. But *it just so happens* that digestion of plant foods in the gut leads to the formation of metabolites that build a healthy immune system,[5] whereas *it just so happens* that metabolites from the digestion of meat are implicated in greater heart disease risk and a compromised immune system.[6, 7] Yes, even with gut microorganisms, meat eaters can't buy a break.

Still, the advocates for a diet based on animal foods continue to vehemently argue their case. Apparently, they believe that while *it just so happens* that the other great apes eat a diet that is 95 to 99 percent plant based (with the occasional treat of insects), we shouldn't allow that fact to challenge our animal-food-based Western diet, as we humans can claim to be some sort of outlying, omnivorous, meat-and-dairy-eating great ape.

Animal food advocates apparently also have no explanation for the fact that humans share all the physical attributes of mammalian herbivores, from dentition, to jaw design and movement, to enzymes in the saliva, to stomach acidity, to intestine length, to the absence of claws, and more. No explanation other than that *it just so happens*, as all these inexplicable similarities represent no more than surprising, senseless happenstance to those who want us to eat flesh as if we were carnivores and consume bovine or caprine mammary secretions as if we were, well, cows or goats.

Oddly, *it just so happens* that the foods that people most often choke on are fish and meat.[8] And *it just so happens* that the foods that most often cause food poisoning are animal foods.[9] Still, fruits and vegetables do indeed sometimes bring on food poisoning, and when that happens and you learn on the news of, say, an *E. coli* outbreak in cucumbers, the cause almost always *just so happens* to turn out to be, not an evil crop of cucumbers, but an animal farm upstream,[10] because *it just so happens* that *E. coli* originates in the colon, and cucumbers don't, as *it just so happens*, have colons.

On a subject crucial to the health of colons, the animal food advocates must find it truly inconvenient that countless new scientific studies keep attributing vital health benefits to fiber, because, after all, *it just so happens* that fiber is found only in plant foods.

And of course, *it just so happens* as well that animal foods bring on inflammation and result in plaque deposits in our arteries, while *it just so happens* that plant foods can reverse that disease process.

Yes, I suppose we can choose to believe that all these things *just so happen*.

Or we can believe that they happen for a reason.

We can then risk an intellectual leap forward by trying to deduce that reason.

Could the reason be that we humans evolved on this Earth primarily as plant eaters, alongside our primarily plant-eating primate cousins? And can we also conclude, given the fact that there are now more than eight billion of us sharing this planet, that it is only by returning to our natural diet of plants that we can protect our own health while giving ourselves, and our fellow creatures, some real hope of allowing life on this planet to become once again sustainable?

Or is it all just wild, inexplicable, freaky bad fortune—one baffling bad break after another—that animal foods bring on so many destructive consequences to our bodies and our planet?

I know which story I believe.

If we are to do our jobs correctly, and move medicine forward, all doctors must now choose which story they believe.

Appendix: Action Plan for Medical Professionals and Members of the Public

Reality Check for Physicians

Doctors: You didn't spend years in medical school just to become another cog in the medical-industrial machine—a system that hands out pills for lifestyle-induced diseases while staying silent about the root causes. If you're not talking to your patients about nutrition, exercise, and real disease prevention, you're not practicing medicine. You're just managing decline.

To avoid being a cog in the machine, here is what you, as a real *disease-reversing doctor,* need to do:

1. **Call out the nonsense in medicine. The next time you see:**

   A cardiology conference sponsored by a bacon company—*say something.*

   A hospital vending machine full of soda and candy—*demand change.*

A colleague saying "diet doesn't matter"—*educate them.*

Silence = complicity. *You are here to lead the charge, not play along.*

2. **Be the doctor you'd want for your own family.** If your own parent, sibling, or child were in that exam room, would you let them believe pills were the only answer? Would you let them keep eating the foods that make them sick without warning them? *Then don't do it to your patients.*
3. **Evaluate the food your hospital or clinic serves to patients.** Does this vital menu promote health or disease? If the latter, consider meeting with the food supervisor to discuss adding healthier options to the food selection. (It often helps to bring a dietitian ally with you.) Many hospitals are now joining the plant-rich menu trend. The food served in the hospital cafeteria to staff and visitors makes a statement about the institute serving it and deserves a similar evaluation and upgrade.
4. **Educate yourself.** Learn about and join the American College of Lifestyle Medicine (lifestylemedicine.org) and the Plantrician Project (plantricianproject.org). With industrial-scale animal agriculture arguably contributing more to global warming than even the burning of fossil fuels, while at the same time driving most deforestation, water depletion, soil erosion, and biodiversity loss, there is a strong ecological imperative for utilizing and promoting plant-predominant diets to your patients and friends. This is humanity's best hope for creating a livable future. Read *Food Is Climate* by my co-author, Glen Merzer, and *Comfortably Unaware* by Richard Oppenlander.
5. **Promote education in applied nutrition** in your practice, hospital, clinic, and community. Hold grand rounds on applied nutrition, bring in guest speakers, do plant-based journal clubs, and have debates on different diet styles. Show "What I Wish I Learned About Nutrition in Medical School"

(movingmedforward.org/general-8). Any of these activities will help foster acceptance that food is a key force in both health and disease.

6. **Write a letter to your state medical board** requesting that a minimum of five hours on diet therapy be made part of the annual continuing medical education (CME) requirements for all newly licensed physicians and for those seeking relicensure.
7. **Mentor** as many medical students, residents, and allied health professionals about applied nutrition as you can. This knowledge should be widespread among the healing professions.
8. **Set a good example** for your patients, your colleagues, your family, and your friends. *Live your best, healthiest, most joyful life.* Eat a plant-predominant diet, walk outside every day, get restorative sleep, avoid alcohol and tobacco use, manage your stress, do some meaningful service every day, spend as much time in nature as you can, and have someone or something in your life that you love.

What Patients and Members of the Public Can Do

Be aware that your doctor's likely ignorance of nutrition is not their fault. The National Board of Medical Examiners ignores the subject of applied nutrition altogether and has no nutrition questions on the National Board exams. This drives a vicious cycle, permitting the medical schools to say, "Until the National Board starts putting nutrition questions on the Board exams, we're not going to clutter up our curriculum with nutrition courses." So the patient's diet as a cause and potential cure of disease remains unmentioned and invisible.

You deserve a nutrition-savvy doctor and it's time our medical schools start producing them! Let the National Board, your state medical board, and your local medical schools know that you demand better from them. Search for a plant-based doctor for yourself at Plantrician.org or LifestyleMedicine.org.

1. **Write or email your state medical boards:** fsmb.org/directory_smb.html. Tell them the average doctor's knowledge of nutrition is woefully inadequate and that you urge the board to include questions on applied nutrition in the National Board examinations, so that medical schools will begin teaching the subject as part of their standard curriculum.
2. **Submit op-eds** to medical journals, major news outlets, or even your local newspaper about the urgent need for nutrition in medical education. Point out that poor diet is the leading cause of preventable death and that incorporating nutrition into medicine reduces healthcare costs.
3. **Write directly to medical schools** you feel connected to (their addresses can be found here: lcme.org/directory/accredited-u-s-programs). Tell them that to maintain your support as a citizen, taxpayer, and consumer of health services, they need to graduate nutritionally aware physicians. Urge them to weave applied nutrition into the basic science teachings in the early years of medical school and throughout the clinical rotations.
4. ***Live your best, healthiest, most joyful life.*** Eat a plant-predominant diet, walk outside every day, get restorative sleep, avoid alcohol and tobacco use, manage your stress, do some meaningful service every day, spend as much time in nature as you can, and have someone or something in your life that you love.
5. **Educate yourself** about plant-based nutrition and consider ways of becoming involved with the plant-based community. Check out the resources that follow, and take advantage of them.

Resources

The following is an admittedly incomplete list of resources; the world of books, guides, websites, and podcasts revolving around plant-strong eating is huge and growing. My apologies to those whose contributions are inadvertently not listed. It was just an oversight! Your contributions are recognized and we appreciate you all!

Quick-Start Guides for Healthy Eating

1. Plantrician Project Quick-Start Guides (adult and pediatric): plantricianproject.org/quickstartguide
2. Physicians Committee for Responsible Medicine 21-Day Vegan Kickstart: kickstart.pcrm.org
3. Rochester Lifestyle Medicine Institute's 15-Day Whole-Food Plant-Based Jumpstart Program (great supportive community—ten CME hours awarded to medical professionals upon completion!): rochesterlifestylemedicine.org/about-jumpstart
4. Dr. McDougall: "How to Start a Plant-Based Diet": drmcdougall.com/education/nutrition/how-to-start-a-plant-based-diet

Not-for-Profit Websites

ClimateHealers.org
FoodIsPower.org
LifestyleMedicine.org
McdougallFoundation.org
NewRootsInstitute.org
NutritionFacts.org
PlantBasedSupport.org
PCRM.org
PlantricianProject.org
RochesterLifestyleMedicine.org
VeganSociety.com
VeganOutreach.org

Other Valuable Websites

BrendaDavisRD.com
ChrisBeatCancer.com
DrBatiste.com
DrEsselstyn.com
DrFuhrman.com
DrMcdougall.com
FoodRevolution.org
ForksOverKnives.com
GoodbyeLupus.com
LivePlantStrong.com
MasteringDiabetes.org
Ornish.com

VeganHealth.org
VegSource.com
VRG.org

Nutrition Studies and Certifications

T. Colin Campbell Center for Nutrition Studies: nutritionstudies.org
Food for Life Instructors: pcrm.org/good-nutrition/plant-based-diets/ffl/become-an-instructor
FoodRevolution.org Plant-Based Coaching Certificate: certificate.foodrevolution.org/join/
Plantrician's Foundations Certificate: plantricianproject.org/plant-based-nutrition-certificate
University of Winchester (UK) six-week online course in plant-based nutrition: winchester.ac.uk/study/further-study-options/cpd/plant-based-nutrition/

Health Coach Directory

plantrician.org/places/category/health-coach/

Podcasts (Available on Most Platforms)

Carleigh Bodrug
Chef AJ
Dr. Columbus Batiste

Dr. McDougall Health and Medical Center
Exam Room Podcast with Chuck Carroll
Glen Merzer Show
Jeff Novick
Nutmeg Notebook
PB with J
Physicians Committee
Plant Based News
Plant Yourself
The Jaroudi Family
The Proof with Simon Hill
The Real Truth About Health
The Rich Roll Podcast
Well Your World

Chefs and Bloggers

Chefaj.com (Chef AJ)
Happyherbivore.com (Lindsay Nixon)
Healthycookingwithshayda.com (Shayda Soleymani)
Kriscarr.com (Kris Carr)
Newthejaroudifamily.com (The Jaroudi Family)
Nutmegnotebook.com (Tami Kramer)
Pbwithj.ca (Jeremy LaLonde)
Plantemus.com (Gustavo Tolosa and Diego Ponieman)
Plantyou.com (Carleigh Bodrug)
Shaneandsimple.com (Shane Martin)
Straightupfood.com (Cathy Fisher)
Wellyourworld.com (Dillon Holmes and Rebecca Reebs)

Authors and Their Books

Neal Barnard, MD, *Dr. Barnard's Program for Reversing Diabetes* and more
Rachel Brown, *For Fork's Sake*
Will Bulsiewicz, MD, *Fiber Fueled*
T. Colin Campbell, PhD, *The China Study* (with Thomas Campbell, MD), *Whole* (with Howard Jacobson), and more
Kris Carr, *Crazy Sexy Diet*
Chef AJ, *The Secrets to Ultimate Weight Loss* and more
Brenda Davis, RD, and Vesanto Melina, RD, *Becoming Vegan* and more
Caldwell Esselstyn, MD, *Prevent and Reverse Heart Disease*
Rip Esselstyn, *The Engine 2 Diet* and more
Joel Fuhrman, MD, *The End of Heart Disease*, *Eat to Live*, and more
Tosia Myers, PhD, and Alan Goldhamer, DC, *Can Fasting Save Your Life?*
Brooke Goldner, MD, *Goodbye Lupus*
Michael Greger, MD, *How Not to Die*, *How Not to Diet*, and more
J. Morris Hicks, *Healthy Eating, Healthy World*, and more
Simon Hill, *The Proof Is in the Plants*
Joanne Kong, PhD, editor, *Vegan Voices*
Alona Pulde, MD, and Matt Lederman, MD, *Wellness to Wonderful* and more
Douglas Lisle, PhD, and Alan Goldhamer, DC, *The Pleasure Trap*
John McDougall, MD, *The Starch Solution* and more
Glen Merzer, *Own Your Health* and more
Victoria Moran, *The Love-Powered Diet* and more
Richard Oppenlander, *Comfortably Unaware*
John Robbins, *Diet for a New America* and more
Ocean Robbins, *31-Day Food Revolution* and more
Rich Roll, *Finding Ultra* and more
Chris Wark, *Chris Beat Cancer*

Cookbook Authors (Low-Fat Vegan Cooking)

Carleigh Bodrug
Chef AJ
Ramses Bravo
Kim Campbell
Ann Crile Esselstyn and Jane Esselstyn
Rip Esselstyn
Cathy Fisher
Ashley Madden
Mary McDougall
Kiki Nelson
Lindsay Nixon
Shayda Soleymani and Gustavo Tolosa
Chef Del Sroufe

Documentaries

Cowspiracy
Eating Our Way to Extinction
Eating You Alive
Fat, Sick and Nearly Dead
Forks Over Knives
I Could Never Go Vegan
PlantPure Nation
Seaspiracy
The Cove
The Game Changers
The Smell of Money
What the Health

Acknowledgments

This book could not have been produced without the unfailing encouragement of my wife, Alese, as well as the stellar efforts of my talented, creative, witty, insightful, and endlessly patient coauthor, Glen Merzer. I shall always be grateful to them both for their contributions.

I thank all the mentors, colleagues, and innovators in the lifestyle medicine movement whose trailblazing of powerful new treatments to reverse disease inspires me on a daily basis.

Thank you to Bruce Sachs for his invaluable graphic contributions to this book.

Glen and I both deeply appreciate the guidance we received from our discerning and diligent editor, Rick Chillot. Rick was ably assisted by Scott Calamar. We also want to thank Leah Wilson and Glenn Yeffeth of BenBella Books for believing in us. Our gratitude goes as well to the whole BenBella team for their steady support and enthusiasm.

Finally, Glen and I want to acknowledge our late friend, teacher, and Bearer of the Light, John Robbins, whose landmark book *Diet for a New America* opened so many eyes and hearts, including our own, to the tragic effects of our current, animal-based diet upon our bodies, upon our fellow creatures caught in the unspeakable factory farm system, and upon our fragile planet itself. We hope this book will help to realize John's vision of a healthier, more joyful world in which humans eat the diet of plants that we were designed by nature to eat.

Notes

Introduction

1. Rakshit S, McGough M. "How does U.S. life expectancy compare to other countries?" Peterson-KFF Health System Tracking. Jan 31, 2025. Accessed May 31, 2025. https://www.healthsystemtracker.org/chart-collection/u-s-life-expectancy-compare-countries/#Life%20expectancy%20at%20birth,%20in%20years,%201980-2023.

Chapter 1

1. Nowadays, we know that antiseptic solutions strong enough to kill germs also kill the cells that line the wound and are needed for healing the laceration. So, in most modern ERs, wounds are washed out with saline solution only.
2. Ellis FR, Sanders TA. "Angina and the Vegan Diet." *American Heart Journal*, Volume 93, Issue 6, 1977:803–805.

Chapter 2

1. Samraj AN et al. "A red meat-derived glycan promotes inflammation and cancer progression." *Proc Natl Acad Sci U S A.* 2015 Jan 13; 112(2):542–7. doi: 10.1073/pnas.1417508112. Epub 2014 Dec 29. PMID: 25548184; PMCID: PMC4299224.
2. Renehan AG et al. "Insulin-like growth factor (IGF)-I, IGF binding

protein-3, and cancer risk: systematic review and meta-regression analysis." Lancet. 2004 Apr 24; 363(9418):1346–53.

3. Erridge C et al. "A high-fat meal induces low-grade endotoxemia: evidence of a novel mechanism of postprandial inflammation." *American Journal of Clinical Nutrition*, Volume 86, Issue 5, 2007:1286–1292. doi: 10.1093/ajcn/86.5.1286.
4. Gatarek P, Kaluzna-Czaplinska J. "Trimethylamine N-oxide (TMAO) in human health." *Excli J.* 2021 Feb 11; 20:301–319. doi: 10.17179/excli2020-3239. PMID: 33746664; PMCID: PMC7975634.
5. Genoni A et al. "Long-term Paleolithic diet is associated with lower resistant starch intake, different gut microbiota composition and increased serum TMAO concentrations." *Eur J Nutr.* 2019. doi: 10.1007/s00394-019-02036-y.
6. Ferro A et al. "Meat intake and risk of gastric cancer in the Stomach cancer Pooling (StoP) project." *Int J Cancer.* 2020 Jul 1; 147(1):45–55. doi: 10.1002/ijc.32707. Epub 2019 Nov 22. PMID: 31584199; PMCID: PMC8550819.
7. Aykan NF. "Red Meat and Colorectal Cancer." Oncol Rev. 2015 Dec 28; 9(1): 288. doi: 10.4081/oncol.2015.288. PMID: 26779313; PMCID: PMC4698595.
8. Orlich MJ et al. "Vegetarian dietary patterns and the risk of colorectal cancers." *JAMA Intern Med.* 2015 May; 175(5):767–76.
9. Torti SV, Manz DH, Paul BT, Blanchette-Farra N, Torti FM. "Iron and Cancer." *Annu Rev Nutr.* 2018 Aug 21; 38:97–125. doi: 10.1146/annurev-nutr-082117-051732. PMID: 30130469; PMCID: PMC8118195.
10. Lan P et al. "High Serum Iron Level Is Associated with Increased Mortality in Patients with Sepsis." *Sci Rep.* 2018 Jul 23; 8(1):11072. doi: 10.1038/s41598-018-29353-2. PMID: 30038422; PMCID: PMC6056487.
11. Gerretsen, I. "You could be swallowing a credit card's weight in plastic every week." CNN. June 17, 2019; https://www.cnn.com/2019/06/11/health/microplastics-ingestion-wwf-study-scn-intl.
12. Skov J et al. "Nematode infections of maricultured and wild fishes in Danish waters: A comparative study." *Aquaculture.* December 2009, 298(1-2):24–28. https://www.sciencedirect.com/science/article/abs/pii/S0044848609008199.
13. Adamidis D, Roma-Giannikou E, Karamolegou K, Tselalidou E, Constantopoulos A. "Fiber intake and childhood appendicitis." *International Journal of Food Sciences and Nutrition.* 51(3), 2000:153–157.

NOTES

Chapter 3

1. For the US: https://www.sca-aware.org/about-sudden-cardiac-arrest/latest-statistics; for Canada: https://www.heartandstroke.ca/what-we-do/media-centre/news-releases/more-cardiac-arrests-are-occurring-and-few-survive
2. Esselstyn CB. "A plant-based diet and coronary artery disease: a mandate for effective therapy." *J Geriatr Cardiol.* 2017 May; 14(5):317–320. doi: 10.11909/j.issn.1671-5411.2017.05.004. PMID: 28630609; PMCID: PMC5466936.
3. Esselstyn CB Jr, Gendy G, Doyle J, Golubic M, Roizen MF. "A way to reverse CAD?" *J Fam Pract.* 2014 Jul; 63(7):356–364b. PMID: 25198208.
4. Ernst E, Pietsch L, Matrai A, Eisenberg J. "Blood rheology in vegetarians." *Br J Nutr.* 1986 Nov; 56(3):555–60. doi: 10.1079/bjn19860136. PMID: 3676231.
5. Mazidi M et al. "Nutrient patterns are associated with discordant apoB and LDL: a population-based analysis." *Br J Nutr.* 2022 Aug 28; 128(4):712–720. doi: 10.1017/S000711452100369X. Epub 2021 Sep 15. PMID: 34523396; PMCID: PMC9346615.
6. Esselstyn, Dr. Caldwell B. *Prevent and Reverse Heart Disease.* Penguin, 2008. p 71.
7. Ajmera, R. "What Is Extra Virgin Olive Oil, & Why Is It Healthy?" Healthline.com. Oct 23, 2023. https://www.healthline.com/nutrition/extra-virgin-olive-oil.
8. Esselstyn CB. "A plant-based diet and coronary artery disease: a mandate for effective therapy." J Geriatr Cardiol. 2017 May; 14(5):317–320. doi: 10.11909/j.issn.1671-5411.2017.05.004. PMID: 28630609; PMCID: PMC5466936.
9. Means, Casey, MD with Calley Means. *Good Energy.* Penguin, 2024. p 84.
10. CDC Diabetes. *National Diabetes Statistics Report 2024.* https://www.cdc.gov/diabetes/php/data-research/index.html.
11. CDC Diabetes. *National Diabetes Statistics Report 2022.* https://www.cdc.gov/diabetes/php/data-research/index.html.
12. American Heart Association. "How Much Sugar Is Too Much?" https://www.heart.org/en/healthy-living/healthy-eating/eat-smart/sugar/how-much-sugar-is-too-much.
13. Gillespie KM, Kemps E, White MJ, Bartlett SE. "The Impact of Free Sugar on Human Health-A Narrative Review." *Nutrients.* 2023 Feb

10; 15(4):889. doi: 10.3390/nu15040889. PMID: 36839247; PMCID: PMC9966020.

14. Sweeney JS. "Dietary Factors That Influence the Dextrose Tolerance Test: A Preliminary Study." *Arch Intern Med* (Chic). 1927 Dec; 40(6):818–830. doi:10.1001/archinte.1927.00130120077005.
15. Jamar G, Pisani LP. "Inflammatory crosstalk between saturated fatty acids and gut microbiota–white adipose tissue axis." *Eur J Nutr* 62, 2023: 1077–1091.
16. Brunzell JD et al. "Improved glucose tolerance with high carbohydrate feeding in mild diabetes." *N Engl J Med.* 1971 Mar 11; 284(10):521–4. doi: 10.1056/NEJM197103112841004. PMID: 5100724; Kiehm TG et al. "Beneficial effects of a high carbohydrate, high fiber diet on hyperglycemic diabetic men." *Am J Clin Nutr.* 1976 Aug; 29(8):895–9. doi: 10.1093/ajcn/29.8.895. PMID: 941870; Anderson JW, Ward K. "High-carbohydrate, high-fiber diets for insulin-treated men with diabetes mellitus." *Am J Clin Nutr.* 1979 Nov; 32(11):2312–21. doi: 10.1093/ajcn/32.11.2312. PMID: 495550.
17. Havel PJ. "A scientific review: the role of chromium in insulin resistance." *Diabetes Educ.* 2004.
18. Barnard ND et al. "A low-fat vegan diet and a conventional diabetes diet in the treatment of type 2 diabetes: a randomized, controlled, 74-wk clinical trial." *Am J Clin Nutr.* 2009 May; 89(5):1588S–1596S. doi: 10.3945/ajcn.2009.26736H. Epub 2009 Apr 1. PMID: 19339401; PMCID: PMC2677007.
19. Chang CC, Lin YT, Lu YT, Liu YS, Liu JF. "Kiwifruit improves bowel function in patients with irritable bowel syndrome with constipation." *Asia Pac J Clin Nutr.* 2010; 19(4):451–7.
20. Appleby PN, Davey GK, Key TJ. "Hypertension and blood pressure among meat eaters, fish eaters, vegetarians and vegans in EPIC–Oxford." *Public Health Nutrition*. 2002; 5(5):645–654. https://www.cambridge.org/core/journals/public-health-nutrition/article/hypertension-and-blood-pressure-among-meat-eaters-fish-eaters-vegetarians-and-vegans-in-epicoxford/678E54EF633FD623EF778BE1BA743C6A; doi:10.1079/PHN2002332.
21. Moore, T. et al. "DASH (Dietary Approaches to Stop Hypertension) Diet Is Effective Treatment for Stage 1 Isolated Systolic Hypertension." *Hypertension*, Volume 38, No. 2, Aug 1, 2001. https://www.ahajournals.org/doi/10.1161/01.HYP.38.2.155.

22. Tomé-Carneiro J, Visioli F. "Plant-Based Diets Reduce Blood Pressure: A Systematic Review of Recent Evidence." *Curr Hypertens Rep.* 2023 Jul; 25(7):127–150. doi: 10.1007/s11906-023-01243-7. Epub 2023 May 13. PMID: 37178356; PMCID: PMC10224875.
23. Indivero, Victoria M., Penn State Research. "Eating lean beef daily can help lower blood pressure" Penn State Research. July 8, 2014. https://www.psu.edu/news/research/story/eating-lean-beef-daily-can-help-lower-blood-pressure.

Chapter 4

1. Starting the FODMAP Diet: https://www.monashfodmap.com/ibs-central/i-have-ibs/starting-the-low-fodmap-diet/; Practical Tips for FODMAP Reintroduction: https://www.monashfodmap.com/blog/practical-tips-fodmap-reintroduction/.
2. Chang CC, Lin YT, Lu YT, Liu YS, Liu JF. "Kiwifruit improves bowel function in patients with irritable bowel syndrome with constipation." *Asia Pac J Clin Nutr.* 2010; 19(4):451–7.
3. Wilkinson-Smith V et al. "Mechanisms underlying effects of kiwifruit on intestinal function shown by MRI in healthy volunteers." *Aliment Pharmacol Ther.* 2019 Mar; 49(6):759–768. doi: 10.1111/apt.15127. Epub 2019 Jan 31. PMID: 30706488; PMCID: PMC6590324.
4. Kano M, Fukudo S, Kanazawa M et al. "Changes in intestinal motility, visceral sensitivity and minor mucosal inflammation after fasting therapy in a patient with irritable bowel syndrome." *Journal of Gastroenterology and Hepatology.* 2006; 21(6):1078–9.
5. Choi HJ et al. "Pro-inflammatory NF-κB and early growth response gene 1 regulate epithelial barrier disruption by food additive carrageenan in human intestinal epithelial cells." *Toxicol. Lett*; 2012 211(3):289–295.
6. Lock JY et al. "Acute exposure to commonly ingested emulsifiers alters intestinal mucus structure and transport properties." *Sci Rep.* 2018; 8:10008.
7. Roberts CL et al. "Translocation of Crohn's disease Escherichia coli across M-cells: contrasting effects of soluble plant fibres and emulsifiers." *Gut.* 2010 Oct; 59(10):1331–9. doi: 10.1136/gut.2009.195370. Epub 2010 Sep 2. PMID: 20813719; PMCID: PMC2976079.
8. Liu Q et al. "Antibacterial and Antifungal Activities of Spices." *Int J Mol Sci.* 2017 Jun 16; 18(6):1283. doi: 10.3390/ijms18061283. PMID: 28621716; PMCID: PMC5486105.

9. O'Mahony, Rachel. *Bioactive Foods in Promoting Health*. Watson Ronald Ross, Preedy Victor R., editors. Academic Press, 2010. p 141–160.
10. Chiba M et al. "Lifestyle-related disease in Crohn's disease: relapse prevention by a semi-vegetarian diet." *World J Gastroenterol.* 2010 May 28; 16(20):2484–95. doi: 10.3748/wjg.v16.i20.2484. PMID: 20503448; PMCID: PMC2877178.
11. Gallagher EJ, LeRoith D. "The proliferating role of insulin and insulin-like growth factors in cancer." *Trends Endocrinol Metab.* 2010 Oct; 21(10):610–8. doi: 10.1016/j.tem.2010.06.007. Epub 2010 Jul 19. PMID: 20663687; PMCID: PMC2949481.
12. Orlich MJ et al. "Vegetarian Dietary Patterns and the Risk of Colorectal Cancers." *JAMA Intern Med.* 2015; 175(5):767–776. doi: 10.1001/jamainternmed.2015.59.
13. O'Keefe SJ et al. "Fat, fibre and cancer risk in African Americans and rural Africans." *Nat Commun.* 2015; 6:6342; O'Keefe SJ et al. "Why do African Americans get more colon cancer than Native Africans?" *J Nutr.* 2007; 137(1 Suppl):175S–182S; Weber C. "Nutrition. Diet change alters microbiota and might affect cancer risk." *Nat Rev Gastroenterol Hepatol.* 2015; 12(6):314; McCarty MF. "Mortality from Western cancers rose dramatically among African-Americans during the 20th century: are dietary animal products to blame?" *Med Hypotheses.* 2001 Aug; 57(2):169–74. doi: 10.1054/mehy.2000.1315. PMID: 11461167.
14. "Making New Connections to Address the Silent Epidemic of Nonalcoholic Fatty Liver Disease." Nat'l Institute of Diabetes and Digestive and Kidney Diseases, NIH. Research Update, Jan 10, 2024. https://www.niddk.nih.gov/news/archive/2024/making-new-connections-address-silent-epidemic-nonalcoholic-fatty-liver-disease.
15. Graffy PM et al. "Automated Liver Fat Quantification at Nonenhanced Abdominal CT for Population-based Steatosis Assessment." *Radiology.* 2019 Nov; 293(2):334–342. doi: 10.1148/radiol.2019190512. Epub 2019 Sep 17. PMID: 31526254; PMCID: PMC6822771.
16. "Fatty liver disease in children is on the rise," Children's Health, accessed 2/13/25, https://www.childrens.com/health-wellness/fatty-liver-disease-in-children-on-the-rise; Yu EL, Schwimmer JB. Epidemiology of Pediatric Nonalcoholic Fatty Liver Disease. Clin Liver Dis (Hoboken). 2021 Apr

13; 17(3):196-199. doi: 10.1002/cld.1027; https://pmc.ncbi.nlm.nih.gov/articles/PMC8043694.C8043694

17. Lufkin, Dr. Robert. *Lies I Taught in Medical School.* BenBella Books, 2024.
18. Li Y et al. "Long-Term Intake of Red Meat in Relation to Dementia Risk and Cognitive Function in US Adults." *Neurology.* Feb 11, 2025, 104 (3).
19. Ornish D et al. "Effects of intensive lifestyle changes on the progression of mild cognitive impairment or early dementia due to Alzheimer's disease: a randomized, controlled clinical trial." *Alz Res Therapy.* 16, 122 (2024).
20. "CNN Documentary Highlights Lifestyle Changes You Can Make to Combat Alzheimer's." US Against Alzheimer's. May 20, 2024. https://www.usagainstalzheimers.org/blog/cnn-documentary-highlights-lifestyle-changes-you-can-make-combat-alzheimers.
21. Natale G, Zhang Y, Hanes DW, Clouston SA. "Obesity in Late-Life as a Protective Factor Against Dementia and Dementia-Related Mortality." *Am J Alzheimers Dis Other Demen.* 2023 Jan–Dec; 38:15333175221111658. doi: 10.1177/15333175221111658. PMID: 37391890; PMCID: PMC10580725.
22. Okereke OI et al., "Dietary fat types and 4-year cognitive change in community-dwelling older women." *Ann Neurol.* 2012 Jul; 72(1):124–34. doi: 10.1002/ana.23593. Epub 2012 May 18. Erratum in: Ann Neurol. 2012 Oct; 72(4):627. PMID: 22605573; PMCID: PMC3405188; Devore EE et al. "Dietary fat intake and cognitive decline in women with type 2 diabetes." *Diabetes Care.* 2009; 32:635–640. doi: 10.2337/dc08-1741.
23. "CNN Documentary Highlights Lifestyle Changes You Can Make to Combat Alzheimer's." US Against Alzheimer's. May 20, 2024. https://www.usagainstalzheimers.org/blog/cnn-documentary-highlights-lifestyle-changes-you-can-make-combat-alzheimers.
24. Testai FD et al, on behalf of the American Heart Association Stroke Council; Council on Cardiopulmonary, Critical Care, Perioperative and Resuscitation; Council on Cardiovascular and Stroke Nursing; and Council on Hypertension. "Cardiac contributions to brain health: a scientific statement from the American Heart Association." Stroke. Volume 55, No. 12, October 10, 2024.
25. LaMotte S. "Common heart conditions raise the risk of dementia, experts say." CNN. Oct. 10, 2024. https://www.cnn.com/2024/10/10/health/heart-dementia-risk-wellness/index.html.

26. Lyman, Howard and Merzer, Glen. *No More Bull!* Simon & Schuster, 2005. p 56.
27. Kim H et al. "Plant-based diets, pescatarian diets and COVID-19 severity: a population-based case–control study in six countries." *BMJ Nutrition, Prevention & Health.* 2021; bmjnph-2021-000272. doi: 10.1136/bmjnph-2021-000272.
28. Merino J et al. "Diet quality and risk and severity of COVID-19: a prospective cohort study." *Gut.* 2021; 70:2096–2104.
29. Albashir AAD. "The potential impacts of obesity on COVID-19." *Clin Med (Lond).* 2020 Jul; 20(4):e109-e113. doi: 10.7861/clinmed.2020-0239. Epub 2020 Jun 22. PMID: 32571783; PMCID: PMC7385759.
30. Ibid.
31. Arulanandam B, Beladi H, Chakrabarti A. "Obesity and COVID-19 mortality are correlated." *Sci Rep.* 13, 5895 (2023). doi:10.1038/s41598-023-33093-3.
32. Masrori P, Van Damme P. "Amyotrophic lateral sclerosis: a clinical review." *Eur J Neurol.* 2020 Oct; 27(10):1918–1929. doi: 10.1111/ene.14393. Epub 2020 Jul 7. PMID: 32526057; PMCID: PMC7540334.
33. Bradley WG, Mash DC. "Beyond Guam: the cyanobacteria/BMAA hypothesis of the cause of ALS and other neurodegenerative diseases." *Amyotroph Lateral Scler.* 2009; 10 Suppl 2:7-20. doi: 10.3109/17482960903286009. PMID: 19929726..
34. Greger, Dr. Michael. *ALS (Lou Gehrig's Disease): Fishing for Answers.* https://nutritionfacts.org/video/als-lou-gehrigs-disease-fishing-for-answers/.
35. Bradley WG, Mash DC. "Beyond Guam: the cyanobacteria/BMAA hypothesis of the cause of ALS and other neurodegenerative diseases." *Amyotroph Lateral Scler.* 2009; 10 Suppl 2:7-20. doi: 10.3109/17482960903286009. PMID: 19929726.
36. Greger, Dr. Michael. *ALS (Lou Gehrig's Disease): Fishing for Answers.* https://nutritionfacts.org/video/als-lou-gehrigs-disease-fishing-for-answers/.
37. Banack SA, Cox PA. "Biomagnification of cycad neurotoxins in flying foxes: implications for ALS-PDC in Guam." *Neurology.* 2003 Aug 12; 61(3):387–9. doi: 10.1212/01.wnl.0000078320.18564.9f. PMID: 12913204.
38. Murch SJ, Cox PA, Banack SA. "A mechanism for slow release of biomagnified cyanobacterial neurotoxins and neurodegenerative disease in Guam." *Proc Natl Acad Sci U S A.* 2004 Aug 17; 101(33):12228–31. doi:

10.1073/pnas.0404926101. Epub 2004 Aug 4. PMID: 15295100; PMCID: PMC514403.

39. Caller TA et al. "A cluster of amyotrophic lateral sclerosis in New Hampshire: a possible role for toxic cyanobacteria blooms." *Amyotroph Lateral Scler.* 2009; 10 Suppl 2:101–8. doi: 10.3109/17482960903278485. PMID: 19929741.
40. Brand LE, Pablo J, Compton A, Hammerschlag N, Mash DC. "Cyanobacterial Blooms and the Occurrence of the neurotoxin beta-N-methylamino-L-alanine (BMAA) in South Florida Aquatic Food Webs." *Harmful Algae.* 2010 Sep 1; 9(6):620–635. doi: 10.1016/j.hal.2010.05.002. PMID: 21057660; PMCID: PMC2968748.
41. Sienko DG, Davis JP, Taylor JA, Brooks BR. "Amyotrophic lateral sclerosis. A case-control study following detection of a cluster in a small Wisconsin community." *Arch Neurol.* 1990 Jan; 47(1):38–41. doi: 10.1001/archneur.1990.00530010046017. PMID: 2294892.
42. Torbick N et al. "Assessing Cyanobacterial Harmful Algal Blooms as Risk Factors for Amyotrophic Lateral Sclerosis." *Neurotoxicity Research.* January 2018 33(1):1–14. doi: 10.1007/s12640-017-9740-y.
43. Masseret E et al. French Network on ALS Clusters Detection and Investigation. "Dietary BMAA exposure in an amyotrophic lateral sclerosis cluster from southern France." *PLoS One.* 2013 Dec 13; 8(12):e83406. doi: 10.1371/journal.pone.0083406. PMID: 24349504; PMCID: PMC3862759.
44. Field NC et al. "Linking β-methylamino-L-alanine exposure to sporadic amyotrophic lateral sclerosis in Annapolis, MD." *Toxicon.* 2013 Aug; 70:179–83. doi: 10.1016/j.toxicon.2013.04.010. Epub 2013 May 6. PMID: 23660330.
45. Rush T, Liu X, Lobner D. "Synergistic toxicity of the environmental neurotoxins methylmercury and β-N-methylamino-L-alanine." *Neuroreport.* 2012 Mar 7; 23(4):216-9. doi: 10.1097/WNR.0b013e32834fe6d6. PMID: 22314682.

Chapter 5

1. Ruble K. "Read the Surgeon General's 1964 Report on Smoking and Health." PBS.org. *Health.* Jan. 12, 2014. https://www.pbs.org/newshour/health/first-surgeon-general-report-on-smokings-health-effects-marks-50-year-anniversary. Accessed Aug. 7, 2025.

2. Leong K, MD. "What's the Deal with McDonald's in Hospitals?" *Medium.* Jan. 22, 2023. https://medium.com/midform/whats-the-deal-with-mcdonald-s-in-hospitals-a4cc989bdac4.
3. Barnett KG. "Physician obesity: the tipping point." *Glob Adv Health Med.* 2014 Nov; 3(6):8–10. doi: 10.7453/gahmj.2014.061. PMID: 25568827; PMCID: PMC4268640, citing Beck M., "Checking up on the doctor: what patients can learn from the way physicians take care of themselves." *The Wall Street Journal.* May 25, 2010. http://online.wsj.com/articles/SB10001424052748704113504575264364125574500.
4. Berry AC et al. "Physician Body Mass Index and Bias Toward Obesity Documentation Patterns." *Ochsner Journal.* 2018 Spring; 18(1):66–71. PMID: 29559873; PMCID: PMC5855427.
5. Ibid.
6. Morgenstern S, Redwood M, Herby A. "An Innovative Program for Hospital Nutrition." *American Journal of Lifestyle Medicine.* 2024; 19(2):320–323. doi: 10.1177/15598276241283158.
7. U.S. Health Insurance Industry Analysis Report, Nat'l Association of Insurance Commissioners, 2023 Mid-Year Report. https://content.naic.org/sites/default/files/industry-analysis-report-2023-health-mid-year.pdf. Accessed Nov. 9, 2024.
8. Vankar P. "Total Revenue of Elevance Health, 2010-2023." July 9, 2025. https://www.statista.com/statistics/214529/total-revenue-of-wellpoint/#:~:text=The%20revenue%20of%20Elevance%20Health,Inc%20on%20June%2028%2C%202022.
9. Zeraatkar D et al. "Red and Processed Meat Consumption and Risk for All-Cause Mortality and Cardiometabolic Outcomes: A Systematic Review and Meta-analysis of Cohort Studies." *Ann Intern Med.* 2019; 171:703–710. Epub 1 October 2019. doi: 10.7326/M19-0655.
10. Ibid.

Chapter 6

1. "McGovern, Buchanan Leading Push for Better Nutrition Education at Medical Schools." Press release of office of Rep. Jim McGovern. Apr. 29, 2024.
2. Ibid.

3. Eisenberg DM et al. "Proposed Nutrition Competencies for Medical Students and Physician Trainees: A Consensus Statement." *JAMA Netw Open*. 2024; 7(9):e2435425. doi:10.1001/jamanetworkopen.2024.35425.
4. Lufkin, Dr. Robert. *Lies I Taught in Medical School*. BenBella Books, 2024. p 273.
5. Means, Casey, MD, with Calley Means. *Good Energy*. Penguin, 2024. p 119.
6. Li, William, MD,. *Eat to Beat Disease*. Grand Central Publishing, 2019. p xv.
7. Lufkin, op. cit., p 118.
8. Palmer, Christopher M., MD. *Brain Energy*. BenBella Books, 2022. p 4.
9. Lufkin, op. cit., p 269.
10. Ibid., p 269.
11. Ali KM, Wonnerth A, Huber K, Wojta J. "Cardiovascular disease risk reduction by raising HDL cholesterol—current therapies and future opportunities." *Br J Pharmacol*. 2012 Nov; 167(6):1177–94. doi: 10.1111/j.1476-5381.2012.02081.x. PMID: 22725625; PMCID: PMC3504986.
12. Lufkin, op. cit., p 271.
13. Hale N. "Inuit metabolism revisited: what drove the selective sweep of CPT1a L479?" *Molecular Genetics and Metabolism*. Volume 129, Issue 4, 2020: 255–271.ISSN 1096-7192.
14. Government of Canada, Statistics Canada. Health reports, Volume 19, No. 1. Modified July 17, 2015. Accessed Aug. 8, 2025. https://www150.statcan.gc.ca/n1/pub/82-003-x/2008001/article/10463/4149059-eng.htm#:~:text=Under%20these%20assumptions%2C%20Inuit%20life,65.0%20to%2067.4)%20in%20Nunavut.
15. Batch JT, Lamsal SP, Adkins M, Sultan S, Ramirez MN. "Advantages and Disadvantages of the Ketogenic Diet: A Review Article." *Cureus*. 2020 Aug 10; 12(8):e9639.
16. Patikorn C et al. "Effects of ketogenic diet on health outcomes: an umbrella review of meta-analyses of randomized clinical trials." *BMC Med 21*, 196 (2023).
17. Ayele GM et al. "Is Losing Weight Worth Losing Your Kidney: Keto Diet Resulting in Renal Failure." *Cureus*. 2023 Mar 22; 15(3):e36546. doi: 10.7759/cureus.36546. PMID: 37095796; PMCID: PMC10121483.

18. Garofalo V et al. "Effects of the ketogenic diet on bone health: A systematic review." *Front Endocrinol* (Lausanne). 2023 Feb 2; 14:1042744. doi: 10.3389/fendo.2023.1042744. PMID: 36817595; PMCID: PMC9932495.
19. Hengist A et al. "Ketogenic diet but not free-sugar restriction alters glucose tolerance, lipid metabolism, peripheral tissue phenotype, and gut microbiome: RCT." *Cell Rep Med.* 2024 Aug 20; 5(8):101667. doi: 10.1016/j.xcrm.2024.101667. Epub 2024 Aug 5. PMID: 39106867; PMCID: PMC11384946.
20. Herms N. "Ketogenic diet: What are the risks?" UChicagoMedicine.org. Jan. 3, 2023.
21. Zhu H et al. "Ketogenic diet for human diseases: the underlying mechanisms and potential for clinical implementations." *Sig Transduct Target Ther* 7, 11 (2022).
22. Noto H et al. "Low-carbohydrate diets and all-cause mortality: a systematic review and meta-analysis of observational studies." *PLoS One.* 2013; 8(1):e55030. doi: 10.1371/journal.pone.0055030. Epub 2013 Jan 25. Erratum in: *PLoS One.* 2019 Feb 7; 14(2):e0212203. doi: 10.1371/journal.pone.0212203. PMID: 23372809; PMCID: PMC3555979.
23. Lufkin, op. cit., p 252.
24. Ibid., p 32, emphasis his
25. Ibid., p 242.
26. Ibid., p 272.
27. Ibid..
28. Means, op. cit., emphasis hers, p 131.
29. Ibid., p 132.
30. Ibid., p 131.
31. Ibid.
32. Ibid., p 132.
33. Taubes G. "The Keto Way: What If Meat Is Our Healthiest Diet?" *The Wall Street Journal.* Jan. 29, 2021.
34. Ibid.
35. Ibid.
36. Ibid.
37. Ibid.
38. Lufkin, op. cit., p 242.

39. Hyman, Mark, MD. *The Pegan Diet*. Little, Brown and Company, 2021. p 58.
40. Ibid., p 60–61.
41. Semuels A. "Over 100 Kids Were Illegally Employed in Dangerous Meat-Packing Plant Jobs." *Time*. Feb. 17, 2023. https://time.com/6256728/meatpacking-child-labor/.
42. Brown AW et al. "Diets high in conjugated linoleic acid from pasture-fed cattle did not alter markers of health in young women." *Nutrition Research*, Volume 31, Issue 1, 2011: 33–41. ISSN 0271-5317. doi: 10.1016/j.nutres.2010.12.003. PMID: 21310304.
43. Hyman, op. cit., p 57–58.
44. Ibid., p 63.
45. Ibid., p 63.
46. People for the Ethical Treatment of Animals. "The Organic and 'Free-Range' Myths." PETA—Animals Used for Food. Accessed Aug. 8, 2025. https://www.peta.org/issues/animals-used-for-food/free-range-organic-meat-myths/.
47. Greene J. "Egg lawsuits test the line between puffery and deception." Reuters. Oct. 25, 2024. https://www.reuters.com/legal/litigation/egg-lawsuits-test-line-between-puffery-deception-2024-10-25/.
48. Ibid.
49. Li, William, MD. *Eat to Beat Disease.* Grand Central Publishing, 2019. p 101–103.
50. Ibid., p 104–105.
51. Ibid., p 120–121.
52. Ibid., p 105–120.
53. Ibid., p 124–125.
54. Ibid., p 125.
55. Ibid.
56. Ventura ER et al. "Association of dietary intake of milk and dairy products with blood concentrations of insulin-like growth factor 1 (IGF-1) in Bavarian adults." *Eur J Nutr.* 2020 Jun; 59(4):1413–1420. doi: 10.1007/s00394-019-01994-7. Epub 2019 May 14. PMID: 31089868.
57. Li Y et al. "Fish intake and risk of melanoma in the NIH-AARP diet and health study." *Cancer Causes Control.* 2022 Jul; 33(7):921–928. doi: 10.1007/s10552-022-01588-5. Epub 2022 Jun 9. PMID: 35676377.
58. Li, William, op. cit., p 25.

59. Ibid., p 134–144.
60. Ibid., p 173–176.
61. Ibid., p 194–196.
62. Ibid, p 201–104.
63. Ibid., p 212–215.
64. Ibid., p 247.
65. Key TJ, Appleby PN, Spencer EA, Travis RC, Roddam AW, Allen NE. "Mortality in British vegetarians: results from the European Prospective Investigation into Cancer and Nutrition (EPIC-Oxford)." *Am J Clin Nutr.* 2009 May; 89(5):1613S-1619S. doi: 10.3945/ajcn.2009.26736L. Epub 2009 Mar 18. PMID: 19297458.
66. Rakshit S, McGough M. "How does U.S. life expectancy compare to other countries?" Peterson-KFF Health System Tracking, Jan. 31, 2025. Accessed May 31, 2025. https://www.healthsystemtracker.org/chart-collection/u-s-life-expectancy-compare-countries/#Life%20expectancy%20at%20birth,%20in%20years,%201980-2023.
67. Johnson SR. "Countries With the Longest and Shortest Life Expectancies." *U.S. News.* Dec. 13, 2024.
68. Gorillas in zoos have been known to develop atherosclerosis, but only from an unnatural zoo diet fed to them by humans, combined with limited space to move and stress.
69. Lufkin, op. cit., p 22.
70. Mills Milton, MD. "The Comparative Anatomy of Eating." Plant Based Nation. Nov. 15, 2019. Accessed Jan. 7, 2025. https://drmiltonmillsplantbasednation.com/the-comparative-anatomy-of-eating/.
71. Mills Milton, MD. "Are We Designed to Eat Meat?" Jeff Nelson VegSource. YouTube. https://www.youtube.com/watch?v=kGDYydkvg3E.

Chapter 7

1. Esselstyn CB. "A plant-based diet and coronary artery disease: A mandate for effective therapy." *Journal of Geriatric Cardiology.* 11(4), 2014: 293–298.
2. Barnard N.D et al.. "A low-fat vegan diet improves glycemic control and cardiovascular risk factors in type 2 diabetic patients." *Diabetes Care,* 32(5), 2009: 791–796.
3. Makki K et al. "The impact of dietary fiber on gut microbiota in host health and disease." *Cell Host & Microbe.* 23(6), 2018: 705–715.

4. Turner-McGrievy GM et al. "Comparative effectiveness of plant-based diets for weight loss." *JAMA*. 177(1), 2017: 76–83.
5. Esselstyn CB (2014), op. cit.
6. Ernst E et al. "Blood rheology in vegetarians." *The British Journal of Nutrition*. 56(3), December 1986:555–60.
7. Whelton PK et al. "Sodium, blood pressure, and cardiovascular disease." *Circulation Research*. 122(10), 2018:1562–1575.

Chapter 8

1. Videle J. "Comparison of Farming in Production of Food Per Acre." The Humane Herald. January 3, 2019. https://humaneherald.org/wp-content/uploads/2019/01/production-of-foods-per-acre.pdf.
2. Rao S, Jain A, Shu S. "The lifestyle carbon dividend: assessment of the carbon sequestration potential of grasslands and pasturelands reverted to native forests." American Geophysical Union Fall Meeting, 2015.
3. Weston P. "Forgotten epidemic: with over 280 million birds dead how is the avian flu outbreak evolving." *The Guardian*. Sep. 4, 2024. https://www.theguardian.com/environment/article/2024/sep/04/forgotten-epidemic-with-over-280-million-birds-dead-how-is-the-avian-flu-outbreak-evolving.
4. Salazar CB et al. "Future pandemics might be caused by bacteria and not viruses: Recent advances in medical preventive practice." *Int J Health Sci* (Qassim). 2022 May–Jun; 16(3):1–3. PMID: 35599938; PMCID: PMC9092534.
5. Ali Reza ASM et al. "Mechanistic insight into immunomodulatory effects of food-functioned plant secondary metabolites." *Crit Rev Food Sci Nutr*. 2023; 63(22):5546–5576. doi: 10.1080/10408398.2021.2021138. Epub 2021 Dec 27. PMID: 34955042.
6. American Heart Association. "Chemicals produced in the gut after eating red meat may contribute to heart disease risk." American Heart Association News. Aug. 1, 2022. https://www.heart.org/en/news/2022/08/01/chemicals-produced-in-the-gut-after-eating-red-meat-may-contribute-to-heart-disease-risk.
7. Krieger K. "Meat, Multiple Sclerosis, and the Microbiome; Studying the connections between meat, gut bacteria, and autoimmune attacks on the nervous system." *Uconn Today*. Jan. 27, 2022.
8. Saccomanno S et al. "Risk factors and prevention of choking." *Eur J Transl*

Myol. 2023 Oct 27; 33(4):11471. doi: 10.4081/ejtm.2023.11471. PMID: 37905785; PMCID: PMC10811631.

9. Coyle D. "Top 9 Foods Most Likely to Cause Food Poisoning." Healthline. June 26, 2023.
10. Gill LL. "Ten Risky Recalled Foods You Should Know About." *Consumer Reports.* March 30, 2023.

Index

INDEX

INDEX

INDEX

INDEX

INDEX

About the Authors

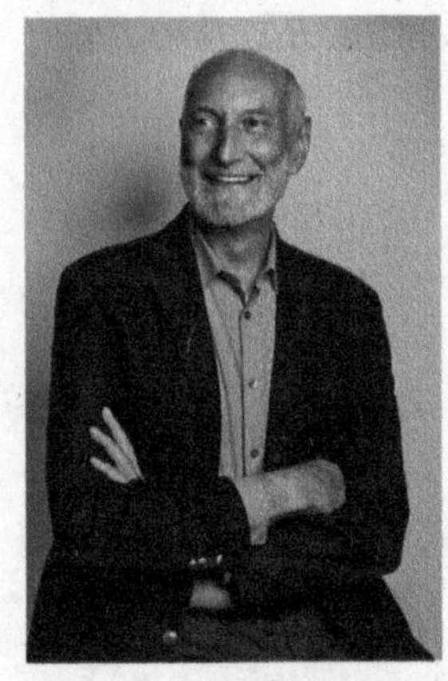

Michael A. Klaper, MD, is a graduate of the University of Illinois College of Medicine in Chicago and has practiced acute care medicine in Hawaii, Canada, California, Florida, and New Zealand. Far more fulfilling to him is his current practice, focusing on health-promoting food and lifestyle choices to arrest and often reverse chronic disease.

To improve his own health and to minimize the suffering of sentient beings, Dr. Klaper adopted a plant-based diet in 1981. Since then, he has promoted the many benefits of plant-predominant nutrition in lectures to medical audiences as well as to the general public across North America and internationally.

Dr. Klaper serves as director of the nonprofit Moving Medicine Forward initiative (movingmedforward.org), dedicated to creating a new generation of nutritionally aware physicians and allied health professionals. He has authored numerous articles on plant-based nutrition and makes the latest information on health and nutrition available through his website, DoctorKlaper.com, where visitors can find the many videos and DVDs he has produced, as well as subscribe to his free newsletter, *The Forward Report*.

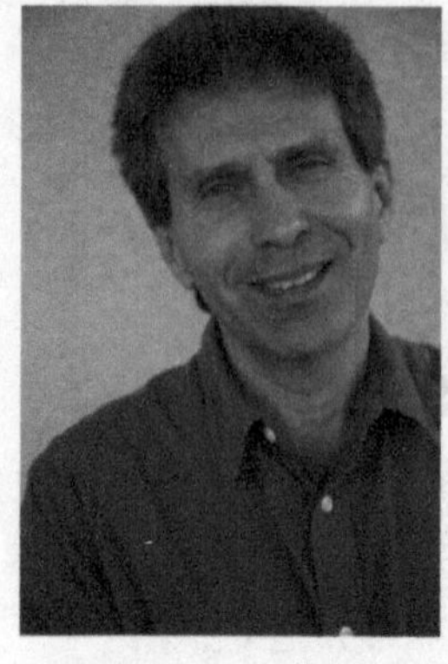

Glen Merzer is a playwright, screenwriter, film director, podcast host, and author. He has authored or co-authored more than a dozen books advocating a diet of whole plant foods. Glen's latest books are *Food Is Climate: A Response to Al Gore, Bill Gates, Paul Hawken, and the Conventional Narrative on Climate Change*; *Own Your Health*; and *America Goes Vegan!* Glen has started a podcast cleverly named *The Glen Merzer Show*, which can be found on YouTube and other podcast platforms. He recently directed his first feature film, *Buddhist Blues*. You can find Glen at GlenMerzer.com.